Drug Interactions Index

SO-BBX-398

Fred Lerman, M.D.
Robert T. Weibert, Pharm.D.

Medical Economics Books
Oradell, New Jersey 07649

Library of Congress Cataloging in Publication Data

Lerman, Fred.
   Drug interactions index.

   Bibliography: p.
   Includes indexes.
   1. Drug interactions.   2. Drug-nutrient
interactions.   I. Weibert, Robert T.   II. Title.
[DNLM: 1. Drug interactions—Handbooks.   QV 38
L616d]
RM302.L47   1982   615'.7045   82-8232
ISBN 0-87489-266-X

Design by Jerry Wilke

ISBN 0-87489-266-X

Medical Economics Company Inc.
Oradell, New Jersey 07649

First Printing   September, 1982
Second Printing   March, 1983

Printed in the United States of America

To our families,
for their help with our work
and their patience during the long period of time
we devoted to this project instead of to them

How to use this book

Finding a specific interaction in *Drug Interactions Index* is a quick, three-step process that takes only a minute or two to master. All you have to know are the trade or generic names of the drugs in question. For example: You want to know if Flagyl (metronidazole) may be safely prescribed for a patient taking Coumadin (warfarin). Here's what to do:

Step 1. Turn to **Section I: Name Index** (blue-edged pages). Look up Flagyl and Coumadin (or metronidazole and warfarin) to find their three-digit *code numbers*. They'll look like this:

by trade names	*OR*	*by generic names*
Flagyl: 384		**metronidazole: 384**
(metronidazole)		(Flagyl)
Coumadin: 568		**warfarin: 568**
(warfarin)		(Athrombin-K, Coumadin, Panwarfin)

(Each drug has been assigned an arbitrary, even-numbered code.)

Step 2. Turn to **Section II: Number Index** (red-edged pages). Find the **384** group of numbers; and scan the list for **568**; or find the **568** group, and scan for **384**. In either case, the *interaction number* for Flagyl and Coumadin, I-299, will follow:

384-108: **I-133**	*OR*	568-288: **I-293**
-140: **I-299**		-302: **I-295**
-166: **I-459**		-344: **I-297**
-232: **I-555**		-366: **I-267**
-568: **I-299**		-384: **I-299**

(Each interaction has been assigned an arbitrary, odd-numbered code.)

Step 3. For the interaction description, turn to **Section III: Interactions** (gray-edged pages), and look for Interaction #I-299. Basically, that's all there is to it.

Additional Features

- **Interaction titles.** When you locate Interaction #I-299, you will find that its title is *not*:

WARFARIN $\longleftrightarrow$ METRONIDAZOLE

568   384

but rather:

ANTICOAGULANTS, $\longleftrightarrow$ METRONIDAZOLE
ORAL

140   742   384
568   744

This is because *other* oral anticoagulants also react as warfarin does with metronidazole. But those other anticoagulants were assigned different code numbers because they do not react identically with drugs *other than* metronidazole. Only drugs that react identically with all other drugs can have identical code numbers.

To convert drug code numbers back into drug names, turn to the **Appendix,** which lists generic names by number and provides information on the clinical orientation of each drug or drug class.

- **Three or more drugs.** At times, you may start out with three or more drugs of interest. If the patient in the example above were also taking Lanoxin (#224), you'd need to check 384-568 (Flagyl-Coumadin), 384-224 (Flagyl-Lanoxin), and 568-224 (Coumadin-Lanoxin) in the Number Index.

But when a number pair does not appear in the Number Index, it means that our current research has not uncovered any significant, adverse interaction between the two drugs involved.

- **Combination products (mixtures).** Products with more than one *active* ingredient are flagged with an "(M)" in the Name Index, and listed like this:

Actifed (M)
pseudoephedrine: **596,**
triprolidine: **756**

Since the activity of a mixture includes the action of each component, all the numbers involved should be used in constructing number pairs to be checked in the Number Index. In the example above, Actifed would have *two* numbers: 596 and 756.

Note: Only *reacting* ingredients are listed for each mixture. For complete lists of mixture ingredients, as well as the most up-to-date information, manufacturers' published data should be checked.

- **CNS depressants.** Drugs with CNS depressant activity are listed in the Name Index with a "D" following their code numbers; for example:

hydromorphone: 840, D
(Dilaudid)

When more than one "D" drug is taken, the depressant effects are additive. See **Interaction #I-435.**

- **Drug-food interactions.** These can be just as significant as drug-drug interactions, and should not be overlooked. Drugs that interact with foods are listed in the Name Index with "F" numbers; for example:

Achromycin: 880, F-16
(tetracycline)

The "F" number (F-16 in the example above) directs you to a specific description in the Food Interactions section, starting on page 260.

For additional details, see the introductory text at the beginning of each section.

Contents

Note to readers

This book was conceived, written, and designed to serve only as a quick, practical guide to significant adverse drug interactions and their clinical implications. Its emphasis is on the essential information that is most helpful to the practicing clinician.

It is not intended to be a comprehensive treatise that explores pharmacologic mechanisms or other background material. Such information is included only when it contributes to proper clinical management. The excellent references listed in the Bibliography are recommended for those interested in further research.

Behind the mathematical simplicity of this book's format lie a number of difficult subjective decisions, such as: which interactions to include, which to exclude; how to interpret conflicting data; when to refer to individual drugs, when to refer to classes; and so on.

After an exhaustive search of currently available data, we included the drug-drug and drug-food interactions that, in our best judgment, are of greatest significance for the practitioner. We deliberately excluded interactions inadequately documented or of dubious importance.

Nevertheless, the reader should not assume that two given drugs do not interact adversely simply because no interaction is listed for them here. Any drug combination should be used with caution, especially since idiosyncratic reactions are always possible.

Adverse effects are, of course, possible even with single-drug therapy. Potential reactions to individual drugs are mentioned here only when they relate to the interaction in question, or to the suggested management or monitoring of the patient during combination therapy. As in any clinical situation involving possibly hazardous treatment, the clinician must exercise his professional responsibility to inform the patient of potential risks.

The suggestions included in each interaction description for treating, minimizing, and preventing adverse effects are summaries of currently preferred methods. They are offered only as guidelines, and must necessarily be adapted according to the individual needs and history of each patient. The clinician actively involved in patient care is in the best position to decide what is right for each case.

Preface

Drug Interactions Index is a practical ready-reference for any health professional involved in drug therapy. It is designed to simplify the flood of often confusing and conflicting clinical data presented to today's beleaguered practitioner. Two notable features make this possible: the book's unique numbering system and the design of the interaction descriptions.

The numbering system, which allows remarkably quick access to needed clinical information, leads the user to any specific drug-drug or drug-food interaction *in seconds*. (See "How to Use This Book," page v, for details.) It also provides instantaneous trade name ⟷ generic name conversion and simplifies the handling of drug classes and combination products.

Each of the 341 interaction descriptions is designed as a concise précis of essential facts, highlighting the information most useful for *actual clinical practice*. Descriptions are supplemented with suggestions for treating, minimizing, and preventing adverse effects.

The multiplicity of drugs in today's armamentarium and the frequency of multiple-drug therapy make the problem of adverse drug interactions more vexing than ever before. It's often been said that it "would take a computer" to keep track of it all. With the computer-like precision of this book's unique numbering system, essential, practical drug interaction data will be easily accessible for the health-care provider.

Publisher's notes

During his more than 35 years in the private practice of urology, Fred Lerman, M.D., F.A.C.S., saw first-hand the overwhelming need for a book "to aid the beleaguered prescriber" in the complex task of managing multiple-drug regimens. This led to his creation of the ingenious drug numbering/indexing system that is the key to this book.

Dr. Lerman is currently Director of Medical Care for Alexian Brothers Hospital in Elizabeth, N.J. He has been Clinical Instructor in Urology at the New York College of Medicine and the New Jersey College of Medicine, President of the Medical Staff and Chief of Urologic Surgery at Elizabeth General Hospital, Chairman of the Urology Section for the New Jersey Medical Society, and has published numerous urological articles in the *Journal of Urology* and the *Journal of the Medical Society of New Jersey*.

Robert T. Weibert, Pharm.D., is Associate Clinical Professor at the University of California, San Francisco, School of Pharmacy, San Diego Program. His specialty is the role of the pharmacist in ambulatory care, particularly in anticoagulation and hypertension therapy. He is the co-author of *Improving Patient Medication Compliance* (Medical Economics Books, 1980). His work has appeared in a number of professional journals, including the *Journal of the American Pharmaceutical Association* and the *American Journal of Hospital Pharmacy*.

Acknowledgments

Many people, in addition to our families, have helped in the development of this book. We would like to acknowledge, with special gratitude, those who contributed specific expertise:

Kevin Cadigan, R.Ph., Barry Cohen, M.D., Burt Eisenbud, David Kaufman, M.D., Larry Kaufman, Joseph Klinger, M.D., Barry Levine, Phil Palmerson Jr., R.Ph., Diane Pelosi, Nancy Semon, Steven Strauss, Pharm.D.

Name Index

HOW TO USE THIS SECTION

The NAME INDEX is STEP 1 in locating an
interaction description (see "How to Use This Book,"
page v). Consult this section to find the three-digit *code
numbers* of the drugs you're interested in.

Every drug can be looked up by either its generic or its
common trade name(s). Generic names are all lower-
case; trade names are capitalized. Corresponding trade
names are listed in parentheses under generic names,
and corresponding generic names under trade names.

For example: You want to look up Flagyl and
Coumadin (or metronidazole and warfarin). They'll look
like this:

by trade names OR *by generic names*

Flagyl: 384
(metronidazole)

Coumadin: 568
(warfarin)

metronidazole: 384
(Flagyl)

warfarin: 568
(Athrombin-K, Coumadin, Panwarfin)

(Each drug has been assigned an arbitrary, even-
numbered code. Drugs that react identically have
identical code numbers.)

Products with more than one *active* ingredient
(mixtures) are flagged with an "(M)" and listed like
this:

Actifed (M)
pseudoephedrine: **596,**
triprolidine: **756**

NOTE: Only *reacting* ingredients are listed for each
mixture. For complete lists of mixture ingredients, as
well as the most up-to-date information, manufacturers'
published data should be checked.

Drugs with CNS depressant activity are listed in this section with a "D" following their code numbers; for example:

hydromorphone: 840, D
(Dilaudid)

When more than one "D" drug is taken, the depressant effects are additive. When dealing with two or more such drugs, see Interaction #I-435 in Section III.

Drug-food interactions can be just as significant as drug-drug interactions, and should not be overlooked. Drugs that interact with foods are listed in this section with "F" numbers; for example:

Achromycin: 880, F-16
(tetracycline)

The "F" number (F-16 in the example above) directs you to a specific description in the FOOD INTERACTIONS section, starting on page 260.

All drug code numbers, "D"s, and "F" numbers are printed in blue in this section.

Once you've found the drug code numbers of interest, proceed to Section II: NUMBER INDEX (red-edged pages).

Accelerase-PB-Caps (M)
atropine: **132,** belladonna: **136,**
calcium carbonate: **726,**
phenobarbital: **434, D**

acetaminophen: 102
(Phenaphen, Tempra, Tylenol)

acetazolamide: 104, D, F-4
(Diamox)

acetohexamide: 826
(Dymelor)

acetophenazine: 848, D
(Tindal)

acetylcholine chloride: 792
(Miochol)

acetyldigitoxin: 804
(Acylanid)

Achromycin: 880, F-16
(tetracycline)

Achromycin V: 880, F-16
(tetracycline)

Achrostatin V (M)
tetracycline: **880, F-16**

ACTH: 200
(corticotropin)

Acthar: 200
(corticotropin)

Actidil: 756, D
(triprolidine)

Actifed (M)
pseudoephedrine: **596,**
triprolidine: **756, D**

Actifed-C Expectorant (M)
codeine: **192, D,** pseudoephedrine:
596, triprolidine: **756, D**

actinomycin D: 106
(Cosmegen)

activated charcoal: 702

Acylanid: 804
(acetyldigitoxin)

Adapin: 888, D
(doxepin)

Adipex-8: 770
(phentermine)

Adipex-P: 770
(phentermine)

Adrenalin: 250
(epinephrine)

Adriamycin: 238
(doxorubicin)

Adroyd: 708
(oxymetholone)

Adrucil: 764
(fluorouracil)

Aerosporin: 450
(polymyxin B sulfate)

Afrin: 876
(oxymetazoline)

Agoral Plain: 832
(mineral oil)

A-HydroCort: 202
(cortisol, hydrocortisone)

Akineton: 736, D
(biperiden)

Albalon-A Liquifilm (M)
naphazoline: **876**

albuterol: 876
(Proventil, Ventolin)

**alcohol (all alcoholic
beverages): 108, D**

Alconefrin: 442
(phenylephrine)

Aldactazide (M)
hydrochlorothiazide: **882, F-8,**
spironolactone: **508, F-8**

Aldactone: 508, F-8
(spironolactone)

Aldoclor (M)
chlorothiazide: **882, F-8,**
methyldopa: **376, D, F-3**

Aldomet: 376, D, F-3
(methyldopa)

Aldoril (M)
hydrochlorothiazide: **882, F-8,**
methyldopa: **376, D, F-3**

Alka-Seltzer (M)
aspirin: **112,** sodium
bicarbonate: **500**

Alka-2: 726, F-17
(calcium carbonate)

alkavervir: 760, F-3
(Veriloid)

Alkeran: 764
(melphalan)

Allerest Tabs (M)
chlorpheniramine: 756, D,
phenylpropanolamine: 444

allobarbital: 772, D
(Diadol)

allopurinol: 110
(Lopurin, Zyloprim)

Alophen: 832
(phenolphthalein)

Alphadrol: 798
(fluprednisolone)

alphaprodine: 840, D
(Nisentil)

alprazolam: 774, D
(Xanax)

alseroxylon: 864, D, F-3
(Rautensin, Rauwiloid)

Alternagel: 722
(aluminum hydroxide)

Alu-Cap: 722
(aluminum hydroxide)

Aludrox (M)
aluminum hydroxide gel: 722,
magnesium hydroxide: 334

aluminum aspirin: 112

aluminum carbonate gel: 722
(Basaljel)

aluminum glycinate: 722

aluminum hydroxide: 722
(Alternagel, Alu-Cap, Alu-Tab,
Amphojel, Columa, Nutrajel)

aluminum phosphate: 722
(Phosphaljel)

Alupent: 592
(metaproterenol)

Alurate: 772, D
(aprobarbital)

Aluscop (M)
dihydroxyaluminum aminoacetate:
722, magnesium hydroxide: 334,
methscopolamine: 374

Alu-Tab: 722
(aluminum hydroxide)

amantadine: 114
(Symmetrel)

ambenonium: 792
(Mytelase)

Ambenyl Expectorant (M)
bromodiphenhydramine: 756, D,
codeine: 192, D,
diphenhydramine: 226, D

Ambodryl: 756, D
(bromodiphenhydramine)

Amcill: 122, F-5
(ampicillin—oral)

Amcill-S: 122
(ampicillin—injection)

Amen: 586
(medroxyprogesterone)

Americaine: 718
(benzocaine)

Amesec (M)
aminophylline: 902, F-12,
amobarbital: 772, D,
ephedrine: 248

Amid-Sal: 866
(salicylamide)

amikacin: 704
(Amikin)

Amikin: 704
(amikacin)

amiloride: 614
(Midamor)

aminobenzoic acid: 116
(Pabagel, Pabanol, PreSun,
Ray-Nox, Sunbrella)

aminophylline: 902, F-12
(Somophyllin)

aminosalicylic acid: 118
(Parasal)

Amitid: 888, D
(amitriptyline)

Amitone: 726, F-17
(calcium carbonate)

Amitril: 888, D
(amitriptyline)

amitriptyline: 888, D
(Amitid, Amitril, Elavil, Endep)

ammonium acid phosphate: 892

ammonium chloride: 892

amobarbital: 772, D
(Amytal)

Amodrine (M)
aminophylline: 902, F-12,
phenobarbital: 434, D,
racephedrine: 248

Apresoline: 296, F-8
  (hydralazine)

Apresoline-Esidrix (M)
  hydralazine: 296, F-8,
  hydrochlorothiazide: 882, F-8

aprobarbital: 772, D
  (Alurate)

AquaMEPHYTON: 898
  (phytonadione, vitamin K₁)

Aquasol E: 540
  (tocopherol, vitamin E)

Aquatag: 882, F-8
  (benzthiazide)

Aquatensen: 882, F-8
  (methyclothiazide)

Aquex: 882, F-8
  (benzthiazide)

Ara-C: 764
  (cytarabine, cytosine arabinoside)

Aramine: 354
  (metaraminol)

Arcylate: 866
  (salsalate)

Arfonad: 760, F-3
  (trimethaphan)

Aristocort: 798
  (triamcinolone)

Arlidin: 896
  (nylidrin)

Artane: 550, D
  (trihexyphenidyl)

Arthrolate: 866
  (sodium thiosalicylate)

Arthropan Liquid: 866
  (choline salicylate)

A.S.A. Compound (M)
  aspirin: 112, caffeine: 146,
  phenacetin: 432

Asbron G (M)
  theophylline: 902, F-12

ascorbic acid: 128
  (Cecon, Cevalin, Cevi-Bid,
  Ce-Vi-Sol, Viterra C)

Ascriptin (M)
  aluminum hydroxide: 722, aspirin:
  112, magnesium hydroxide: 334

Ascriptin with Codeine (M)
  aluminum hydroxide: 722,
  aspirin: 112, codeine: 192, D,
  magnesium hydroxide: 334

Asendin: 888, D
  (amoxapine)

Asma-Lief (M)
  ephedrine: 248, phenobarbital:
  434, D, theophylline: 902, F-12

asparaginase: 130
  (Elspar)

Aspergum: 112
  (aspirin)

aspirin: 112
  (Aspergum, Ecotrin, Empirin,
  Measurin)

Aspirols: 730
  (amyl nitrite)

AsthmaNefrin: 250
  (epinephrine)

Atabrine: 486
  (quinacrine)

Atarax: 298, D
  (hydroxyzine)

atenolol: 776, F-8
  (Tenormin)

Athrombin-K: 568, F-2
  (warfarin)

Ativan: 774, D
  (lorazepam)

Atrocholin (M)
  homatropine: 738

Atromid-S: 186
  (clofibrate)

atropine: 132
  (many trade names
  for eye preparations)

attapulgite: 702

Aureomycin: 880, F-16
  (chlortetracycline)

aurothioglucose: 818
  (Solganal)

AVC (M)
  sulfanilamide: 872

Aventyl: 888, D
  (nortriptyline)

Avlosulfon: 208
  (dapsone)

Azapen: 844
(methicillin)

azatadine: 756, D
(Optimine)

azathioprine: 134
(Imuran)

Azo Gantanol (M)
phenazopyridine: 822,
sulfamethoxazole: 516

Azo Gantrisin (M)
phenazopyridine: 822,
sulfisoxazole: 526

Azolid: 440
(phenylbutazone)

Azolid-A (M)
aluminum hydroxide gel: 722,
magnesium trisilicate: 728,
phenylbutazone: 440

Azo-Mandelamine (M)
methenamine mandelate:
360, F-11, phenazopyridine: 822

Azo-Soxazole (M)
phenazopyridine: 822,
sulfisoxazole: 526

Azo-Sulfstat (M)
phenazopyridine: 822,
sulfamethizole: 514

Azotrex (M)
phenazopyridine: 822,
sulfamethizole: 514,
tetracycline: 880, F-16

Azulfidine: 522
(sulfasalazine)

bacampicillin—oral: 122, F-5
(Spectrobid)

Bacarate: 770
(phendimetrazine)

baclofen: 868, D
(Lioresal)

Bactocill: 410
(oxacillin—injection)

Bactocill: 410, F-5
(oxacillin—oral)

Bactrim (M)
sulfamethoxazole: 516

Banthine: 738
(methantheline)

Barbidonna Elixir, Tabs (M)
atropine: 132, hyoscyamine: 136,
phenobarbital: 434, D,
scopolamine: 492, D

barbital: 772, D

barley malt extract: 832
(Maltsupex)

Basaljel: 722
(aluminum carbonate gel)

Bayer-205: 838
(suramin)

BCG vaccine: 822

BCNU: 158
(BiCNU)

beclomethasone: 798
(Beclovent, Vanceril)

Beclovent: 798
(beclomethasone)

Belap (M)
belladonna: 136,
phenobarbital: 434, D

Belladenal Tabs (M)
belladonna: 136,
phenobarbital: 434, D

**belladonna alkaloids, extract,
leaf, or tincture:** 136

Bellafoline: 136
(levorotatory alkaloids of
belladonna)

Bellergal (M)
belladonna: 136, ergotamine:
812, phenobarbital: 434, D

benactyzine: 738

Benadryl: 226, D
(diphenhydramine)

Bendectin (M)
doxylamine: 756, D,
pyridoxine: 482

bendroflumethiazide: 882, F-8
(Naturetin)

Benemid: 458
(probenecid)

Benisone: 798
(betamethasone)

Benn: 458
(probenecid)

Bricanyl: 598
(terbutaline)

Bristacycline: 880, F-16
(tetracycline)

Bristamycin: 814, F-5
(erythromycin)

bromodiphenhydramine: 756, D
(Ambodryl)

brompheniramine: 756, D
(Dimetane)

Bronchobid Duracaps (M)
ephedrine: **248,**
theophylline: **902, F-12**

Brondecon (M)
oxtriphylline: **902, F-12**

Bronkephrine: 602
(ethylnorepinephrine)

Bronkodyl: 902, F-12
(theophylline)

Bronkolixir (M)
ephedrine: **248,** phenobarbital:
434, D, theophylline: **902, F-12**

Bronkometer: 604
(isoetharine)

Bronkosol: 604
(isoetharine)

Bucladin-S: 756, D
(buclizine)

buclizine: 756, D
(Bucladin-S)

Bufferin (M)
aluminum glycinate: **722,**
aspirin: **112,**
magnesium carbonate: **332**

busulfan: 144
(Myleran)

butabarbital: 772, D
(Buticaps, Butisol)

butacaine: 718
(Butyn)

butalbital: 772, D
(Sandoptal)

butaperazine: 848, D
(Repoise)

Butatrax (M)
amobarbital: **772, D,**
butabarbital: **772, D**

Butazolidin: 440
(phenylbutazone)

Butazolidin Alka (M)
aluminum hydroxide gel: **722,**
magnesium trisilicate: **728,**
phenylbutazone: **440**

Butibel (M)
belladonna: **136,**
butabarbital: **772, D**

Butibel-Zyme (M)
belladonna: **136,**
butabarbital: **772, D**

Buticaps: 772, D
(butabarbital)

Butisol: 772, D
(butabarbital)

butorphanol: 840, D
(Stadol)

Butyn: 718
(butacaine)

Cafergot P-B Tablets,
Suppositories (M)
belladonna: **136,** caffeine: **146,**
ergotamine: **812,**
pentobarbital: **430, D**

Cafergot Tablets,
Suppositories (M)
caffeine: **146,** ergotamine: **812**

caffeine: 146
(No Doz, Pep-Aid, Stim-Tabs,
Vivarin)

Calan: 910
(verapamil)

Calcidrine Syrup (M)
calcium iodide: **828,**
codeine: **192, D**

calcium carbaspirin: 112
(Calurin)

calcium carbonate: 726, F-17
(Alka-2, Amitone, Chooz,
Dicarbosil, Titralac, Trialka
Tablets, Tums)

calcium chloride: 778

calcium gluceptate: 778

calcium gluconate: 778

calcium iodide: 828

calcium lactate: 778

Calpas (M)
aminosalicylic acid: 118,
isoniazid: 310, F-4,
pyridoxine: 482

Calurin: 112
(calcium carbaspirin)

calusterone: 712
(Methosarb)

Cama Inlay-Tabs (M)
aluminum hydroxide gel: 722,
aspirin: 112,
magnesium hydroxide: 334

Camalox (M)
aluminum hydroxide: 722,
calcium carbonate: 726,
magnesium hydroxide: 334

camphorated tincture of
opium: 752, D
(Paregoric)

Cantil: 738
(mepenzolate)

Cantil with Phenobarbital (M)
mepenzolate: 738,
phenobarbital: 434, D

Capastat: 148
(capreomycin)

Capoten: 616, F-18
(captopril)

capreomycin: 148
(Capastat)

captopril: 616, F-18
(Capoten)

Carafate: 620
(sucralfate)

caramiphen: 736, D

carbamazepine: 150, D, F-1
(Tegretol)

carbenicillin—injection: 152
(Geopen, Pyopen)

carbenicillin—oral: 152, F-5
(Geocillin)

carbenoxolone: 154, F-3, F-8
(Duogastrone)

carbetapentane: 736, D

carbinoxamine: 756, D
(Clistin)

Carbrital Kapseals (M)
carbromal: 582, D,
pentobarbital: 430, D

carbromal: 582, D

Cardilate: 730
(erythrityl tetranitrate)

Cardilate-P (M)
erythrityl tetranitrate: 730,
phenobarbital: 434, D

Cardioquin: 862, F-14
(quinidine)

Cardrase: 782, D
(ethoxzolamide)

carisoprodol: 156, D
(Rela, Soma)

carmustine: 158
(BiCNU)

carphenazine: 848, D
(Proketazine)

Cartrax (M)
hydroxyzine: 298, D,
pentaerythritol tetranitrate: 730

cascara sagrada: 832
(Cas-Evac)

Cas-Evac: 832
(cascara sagrada)

castor oil: 832

Catapres: 190, D, F-3
(clonidine)

CCNU: 764
(CeeNU)

Cebral: 896
(ethaverine)

Ceclor: 788
(cefaclor)

Cecon: 128
(ascorbic acid, vitamin C)

Cedilanid: 804
(lanatoside C)

Cedilanid-D: 804
(deslanoside)

CeeNU: 764
(lomustine)

cefaclor: 788
(Ceclor)

cefadroxil: 788
(Duricef, Ultracef)

Cefadyl: 788
(cephapirin)

cefamandole: 618
(Mandol)

cefazolin: 788
(Ancef, Kefzol)

cefotaxime: 788
(Claforan)

cefoxitin: 788
(Mefoxin)

Celbenin: 844
(methicillin)

Celestone: 798
(betamethasone)

Celontin: 870, D
(methsuximide)

cephalexin: 788
(Keflex)

cephaloglycin: 788
(Kafocin)

cephaloridine: 160
(Loridine)

cephalothin: 162
(Keflin)

cephapirin: 788
(Cefadyl)

cephradine: 164
(Anspor, Velosef)

Cerespan: 418
(papaverine)

Cerose Compound (M)
acetaminophen: 102,
chlorpheniramine: 756, D,
dextromethorphan: 212,
phenylephrine: 442

Cerose DM (M)
dextromethorphan: 212,
phenindamine: 756, D,
phenylephrine: 442

Cerubidine: 764
(daunorubicin)

Cevalin: 128
(ascorbic acid, vitamin C)

Cevi-Bid: 128
(ascorbic acid, vitamin C)

Ce-Vi-Sol: 128
(ascorbic acid, vitamin C)

Chardonna-2 (M)
belladonna: 136,
phenobarbital: 434, D

Chel-Iron: 830
(ferrocholinate)

Chemestrogen: 816
(benzestrol)

Cheracol D Cough Syrup (M)
dextromethorphan: 212

chloral betaine: 790, D
(Beta-Chlor)

chloral hydrate: 790, D
(Noctec, Somnos)

chlorambucil: 764
(Leukeran)

chloramphenicol: 166
(Chloromycetin, Mychel)

chlordiazepoxide: 168, D
(Libritabs, Librium)

chlormezanone: 780, D
(Trancopal)

Chlorohist: 756, D
(chlorpheniramine)

Chloromycetin: 166
(chloramphenicol)

chlorothiazide: 882, F-8
(Diuril)

chlorotrianisene: 816
(TACE)

chlorphenesin: 170, D
(Maolate)

chlorpheniramine: 756, D
(Chlorohist, Chlor-Trimeton,
Histaspan, Teldrin)

chlorphenoxamine: 172, D
(Phenoxene)

chlorphentermine: 770
(Pre-Sate)

chlorpromazine: 174, D
(Thorazine)

chlorpropamide: 176
(Diabinese)

chlorprothixene: 884, D
(Taractan)

chlortetracycline: 880, F-16
(Aureomycin)

chlorthalidone: 882, F-8
(Hygroton)

Chlor-Trimeton: 756, D
(chlorpheniramine)

Chlor-Trimeton Decongestant (M)
chlorpheniramine: 756, D,
pseudoephedrine: 596

chlorzoxazone: 868, D
(Paraflex)

Cholan-HMB Tabs (M)
homatropine: 738,
phenobarbital: 434, D

Choledyl: 902, F-12
(oxtriphylline)

cholestyramine: 178
(Cuemid, Questran)

choline salicylate: 866
(Arthropan Liquid)

Choloxin: 214, F-15
(dextrothyroxine)

Chooz: 726, F-17
(calcium carbonate)

Chromagen Caps (M)
iron: 830

cimetidine: 180
(Tagamet)

Cin-Quin: 862, F-14
(quinidine)

cisplatin: 182
(Platinol)

Claforan: 788
(cefotaxime)

clemastine: 756, D
(Tavist)

Cleocin: 184
(clindamycin)

clidinium: 738
(Quarzan)

clindamycin: 184
(Cleocin)

Clinoril: 606
(sulindac)

Clistin: 756, D
(carbinoxamine)

clofibrate: 186
(Atromid-S)

clonazepam: 188, D
(Clonopin)

clonidine: 190, D, F-3
(Catapres)

Clonopin: 188, D
(clonazepam)

Clopane: 878
(cyclopentamine)

clorazepate: 774, D
(Tranxene)

clortermine: 770
(Voranil)

cloxacillin: 846, F-5
(Cloxapen, Tegopen)

Cloxapen: 846, F-5
(cloxacillin)

Coco-Quinine: 862, F-14
(quinine)

codeine: 192, D

Codimal DH (M)
hydrocodone: 840, D,
phenylephrine: 442,
pyrilamine: 756, D

Codone: 840, D
(hydrocodone)

Cogentin: 736, D
(benztropine)

Colace: 832
(dioctyl sodium sulfosuccinate,
docusate)

ColBENEMID (M)
probenecid: 458

Colestid: 194
(colestipol)

colestipol: 194
(Colestid)

colistimethate: 196
(Coly-Mycin M)

colistin: 198
(Coly-Mycin S)

Colonaid (M)
atropine: 132,
diphenoxylate: 228, D

Colrex Compound (M)
acetaminophen: 102,
chlorpheniramine: 756, D,
codeine: 192, D,
phenylephrine: 442

Darbid: 312
  (isopropamide iodide)

Daricon: 738
  (oxyphencyclimine)

Daricon-PB Tabs (M)
  oxyphencyclimine: 738,
  phenobarbital: 434, D

Darvocet-N 50, 100 (M)
  acetaminophen: 102,
  propoxyphene: 474, D

Darvon: 474, D
  (propoxyphene)

Darvon Compound-65 (M)
  aspirin: 112, caffeine: 146,
  phenacetin: 432,
  propoxyphene: 474, D

Darvon-N: 474, D
  (propoxyphene)

Darvon-N with A.S.A. (M)
  aspirin: 112,
  propoxyphene: 474, D

Darvon with A.S.A. (M)
  aspirin: 112,
  propoxyphene: 474, D

Daserol: 868, D
  (mephenesin)

daunorubicin: 764
  (Cerubidine)

Daxolin: 330, D
  (loxapine)

Deaner: 786
  (deanol)

deanol: 786
  (Deaner)

Deapril-ST (M)
  ergot alkaloids,
  dihydrogenated: 812

Decadron: 798
  (dexamethasone)

Deca-Durabolin: 708
  (nandrolone)

decamethonium: 800
  (Syncurine)

Decapryn: 756, D
  (doxylamine)

Declomycin: 880, F-16
  (demeclocycline)

Declostatin Caps, Tabs (M)
  demeclocycline: 880, F-16

Deconamine (M)
  chlorpheniramine: 756, D,
  pseudoephedrine: 596

Degest (M)
  phenylephrine: 442

Dehist Caps (M)
  chlorpheniramine: 756, D,
  phenylephrine: 442,
  phenylpropanolamine: 444

Deladumone Injection (M)
  estradiol: 816, testosterone: 712

Delalutin: 860
  (hydroxyprogesterone)

Delatestryl: 712
  (testosterone)

Delaxin: 364, D
  (methocarbamol)

Delcid (M)
  aluminum hydroxide: 722,
  magnesium hydroxide: 334

Delestrogen: 816
  (estradiol)

Delta-Cortef: 798
  (prednisolone)

Delta-Dome: 798
  (prednisone)

Deltasone: 798
  (prednisone)

Deltra: 798
  (prednisone)

Demazin (M)
  chlorpheniramine: 756, D,
  phenylephrine: 442

demeclocycline: 880, F-16
  (Declomycin)

Demerol: 346, D
  (meperidine)

Demerol APAP (M)
  acetaminophen: 102,
  meperidine: 346, D

Demi-Regroton (M)
  chlorthalidone: 882, F-8,
  reserpine: 864, D, F-3

Demulen (M)
  ethinyl estradiol: 816,
  ethynodiol diacetate: 860

Dendrid: 838
  (idoxuridine)

Diutensen (M)
cryptenamine: 760, F-3,
methyclothiazide: 882, F-8

Diutensen-R (M)
methyclothiazide: 882, F-8,
reserpine: 864, D, F-3

dobutamine: 876
(Dobutrex)

Dobutrex: 876
(dobutamine)

Doca: 210
(desoxycorticosterone)

docusate: 832
(Colace)

Dolene: 474, D
(propoxyphene)

Dolene AP-65 (M)
acetaminophen: 102,
propoxyphene: 474, D

Dolene Compound-65 (M)
aspirin: 112, caffeine: 146,
phenacetin: 432,
propoxyphene: 474, D

Dolophine: 356, D
(methadone)

Doloral (M)
aminobenzoic acid 116, aspirin:
112, phenobarbital: 434, D

Donnagel (M)
atropine: 132, hyoscine: 492, D,
hyoscyamine: 136,
kaolin-pectin: 702

Donnagel-PG (M)
atropine: 132, hyoscine: 492, D,
hyoscyamine: 136, kaolin-pectin:
702, opium: 752, D

Donnatal Caps, Tabs (M)
atropine: 132, hyoscine: 492, D,
hyoscyamine: 136,
phenobarbital: 434, D

Donnazyme (M)
atropine: 132, hyoscine: 492, D,
hyoscyamine: 136,
phenobarbital: 434, D

dopamine: 234
(Intropin)

Dopar: 320, F-9
(levodopa)

Dopram: 236
(doxapram)

**Dorcol Pediatric Cough
Syrup (M)**
dextromethorphan: 212,
phenylpropanolamine: 444

Doriden: 282, D
(glutethimide)

Dormethan: 212
(dextromethorphan)

doxapram: 236
(Dopram)

doxepin: 888, D
(Adapin, Sinequan)

doxorubicin: 238
(Adriamycin)

Doxychel: 240, F-16
(doxycycline)

doxycycline: 240, F-16
(Doxychel, Vibramycin)

doxylamine: 756, D
(Decapryn)

Dralserp (M)
hydralazine: 296, F-8,
reserpine: 864, D, F-3

Dralzine: 296, F-8
(hydralazine)

Dramamine: 756, D
(dimenhydrinate)

Dristan Caps (M)
aspirin: 112, caffeine: 146,
chlorpheniramine: 756, D,
phenylpropanolamine: 444

Dristan Tabs (M)
aspirin: 112, caffeine: 146,
chlorpheniramine: 756, D,
phenylephrine: 442

Dristan-AF (M)
acetaminophen: 102, caffeine: 146,
chlorpheniramine: 756, D,
phenylephrine: 442

Dristan Cough Formula (M)
chlorpheniramine. 756, D,
dextromethorphan: 212,
phenylephrine: 442

Dristan Time Caps (M)
aluminum hydroxide: 722,
aspirin: 112, caffeine: 146,
magnesium carbonate: 332,
phenindamine: 756, D,
phenylephrine: 442

Drixoral (M)
dexbrompheniramine: 756, D,
pseudoephedrine: 596

Drolban: 712
(dromostanolone)

dromostanolone: 712
(Drolban)

droperidol: 242, D
(Inapsine)

DTIC-Dome: 764
(dacarbazine)

Dulcolax: 832
(bisacodyl)

Duogastrone: 154, F-3, F-8
(carbenoxolone)

Duolax: 832
(danthron)

Duo-Medihaler (M)
isoproterenol: 314,
phenylephrine: 442

Duotrate: 730
(pentaerythritol tetranitrate)

Duphaston: 860
(dydrogesterone)

Durabolin: 708
(nandrolone)

Duracillin A.S.: 844
(penicillin G procaine)

Duraquin: 862, F-14
(quinidine)

Durasal: 866
(magnesium salicylate)

Duricef: 788
(cefadroxil)

Duvoid: 580
(bethanechol)

DV: 816
(dienestrol)

Dyazide (M)
hydrochlorothiazide: 882, F-8,
triamterene: 546, F-3

Dycill: 846, F-5
(dicloxacillin)

dydrogesterone: 860
(Duphaston, Gynorest)

Dymelor: 826
(acetohexamide)

Dynapen: 846, F-5
(dicloxacillin)

dyphylline: 902, F-12
(Dilor, Lufyllin, Neophyl)

Dyprin: 362
(methionine)

Dyrenium: 546, F-3
(triamterene)

Dyspas: 220
(dicyclomine)

E-Carpine (M)
epinephrine: 250

Echodide: 244
(echothiophate)

echothiophate: 244
(Echodide, Phospholine Iodide)

Ecotrin: 112
(aspirin)

Ectasule Minus III: 248
(ephedrine)

Edecrin: 254, F-3
(ethacrynic acid)

edrophonium: 246
(Tensilon)

E.E.S.: 814, F-5
(erythromycin)

E-Ferol: 540
(tocopherol, vitamin E)

Efudex: 764
(fluorouracil)

E-Ionate P.A.: 816
(estradiol)

Elavil: 888, D
(amitriptyline)

Elixicon: 902, F-12
(theophylline)

Elixophyllin: 902, F-12
(theophylline)

Elixophyllin-KI Elixir (M)
potassium iodide: 828,
theophylline: 902, F-12

Elspar: 130
(asparaginase)

Empirin: 112
(aspirin)

Empirin with Codeine (M)
aspirin: 112, codeine: 192, D

E-Mycin: 814, F-5
(erythromycin)

Enarax Tabs (M)
hydroxyzine: 298, D,
oxyphencyclimine: 738

Endal (M)
chlorpheniramine: 756, D,
phenylephrine: 442

Endal Expectorant (M)
chlorpheniramine: 756, D,
codeine: 192, D,
phenylephrine: 442,
phenylpropanolamine: 444

Endep: 888, D
(amitriptyline)

Enduron: 882, F-8
(methyclothiazide)

Enduronyl (M)
deserpidine: 864, D, F-3,
methyclothiazide: 882, F-8

enflurane: 716, D
(Ethrane)

Enovid (M)
mestranol: 816,
norethynodrel: 860

Enovid-E (M)
mestranol: 816,
norethynodrel: 860

Entex (M)
phenylephrine: 442,
phenylpropanolamine: 444

ephedrine: 248
(Ectasule Minus III)

Epicar with Epinephrine (M)
epinephrine: 250

E-Pilo (M)
epinephrine: 250

epinephrine: 250
(Adrenalin, AsthmaNefrin,
Sus-Phrine, Vaponefrin)

Epsom salts: 834
(magnesium sulfate—oral)

Equagesic (M)
aspirin: 112, ethoheptazine:
840, D, meprobamate: 348, D

Equanil: 348, D
(meprobamate)

Ergocaf (M)
caffeine: 146, ergotamine: 812

Ergomar: 812
(ergotamine)

ergonovine: 812
(Ergotrate)

Ergostat: 812
(ergotamine)

ergot alkaloids: 812

ergotamine: 812
(Ergomar, Ergostat, Gynergen)

Ergotrate: 812
(ergonovine)

Erypar: 814, F-5
(erythromycin)

erythrityl tetranitrate: 730
(Cardilate)

Erythrocin: 814, F-5
(erythromycin)

erythromycin: 814, F-5
(Bristamycin, E.E.S., E-Mycin,
Erypar, Erythrocin, Ethril, Ilotycin,
Pediamycin, Pfizer-E, Robimycin,
RP-Mycin)

erythromycin estolate: 252, F-5
(Ilosone)

**erythromycin
lactobionate:** 814, F-5

Esgic (M)
acetaminophen: 102, butalbital:
772, D, caffeine: 146

Esidrix: 882, F-8
(hydrochlorothiazide)

Esimil (M)
guanethidine: 820, F-3,
hydrochlorothiazide: 882, F-8

Eskabarb: 434, D
(phenobarbital)

Eskalith: 326, F-10
(lithium)

Eskatrol (M)
dextroamphetamine: 706,
prochlorperazine: 466, D

esterified estrogens: 816
(Evex, Menest)

Estinyl: 816
(ethinyl estradiol)

Estrace: 816
(estradiol)

estradiol: 816
(Delestrogen, Depo-Estradiol,
E-Ionate P.A., Estrace, Progynon)

Estratest (M)
esterified estrogens: 816,
methyltestosterone: 712

estrogens, conjugated: 816
(Premarin)

estrogens, esterified: 816
(Evex, Menest)

estrone: 816
(Follestrol, Ogen, Theelin,
Theelin R-P)

Estrovis: 816
(quinestrol)

ethacrynic acid: 254, F-3
(Edecrin)

Ethamide: 782, D
(ethoxzolamide)

Ethaquin: 896
(ethaverine)

Ethatab: 896
(ethaverine)

ethaverine: 896
(Cebral, Ethaquin, Ethatab,
Pavaspan)

ethchlorvynol: 256, D
(Placidyl)

ether: 716, D

ethinamate: 258, D
(Valmid)

ethinyl estradiol: 816
(Estinyl, Feminone, Lynoral)

ethionamide: 822
(Trecator-SC)

ethisterone: 860
(Progestalets, Progestoral)

Ethobral (M)
butabarbital: 772, D,
phenobarbital: 434, D,
secobarbital: 494, D

ethoheptazine: 840, D
(Zactane)

ethopropazine: 260, D
(Parsidol)

ethosuximide: 870, D
(Zarontin)

ethotoin: 824, D
(Peganone)

ethoxzolamide: 782, D
(Cardrase, Ethamide)

Ethrane: 716, D
(enflurane)

Ethril: 814, F-5
(erythromycin)

ethylestrenol: 708
(Maxibolin)

ethylnorepinephrine: 602
(Bronkephrine)

ethynodiol diacetate: 860

Etrafon (M)
amitriptyline: 888, D,
perphenazine: 848, D

Euthroid: 886, F-15
(liotrix)

Eutonyl: 836, F-6
(pargyline)

Eutron Filmtabs (M)
methyclothiazide: 882, F-8,
pargyline: 836, F-6

Evex: 816
(esterified estrogens)

Excedrin Caps, Tabs (M)
acetaminophen: 102, aspirin: 112,
caffeine: 146

Excedrin P.M. (M)
acetaminophen: 102,
pyrilamine: 756, D

Ex-Lax: 832
(phenolphthalein)

Exna: 882, F-8
(benzthiazide)

Exna-R (M)
benzthiazide: 882, F-8,
reserpine: 864, D, F-3

Fastin: 770
(phentermine)

Feen-A-Mint: 832
(phenolphthalein)

Femcaps (M)
acetaminophen: 102,
atropine: 132, caffeine: 146,
ephedrine: 248

Feminone: 816
  (ethinyl estradiol)

fenfluramine: 262, D
  (Pondimin)

fenoprofen: 762
  (Nalfon)

fentanyl: 264, D
  (Sublimaze)

Feosol: 830
  (ferrous sulfate)

Feostat: 830
  (ferrous fumarate)

Ferancee (M)
  ascorbic acid: 128,
  ferrous fumarate: 830

Fergon: 830
  (ferrous gluconate)

Fer-in-Sol: 830
  (ferrous sulfate)

Fermalox (M)
  aluminum hydroxide: 722,
  ferrous sulfate: 830,
  magnesium hydroxide: 334

Fero-Folic 500 (M)
  ascorbic acid: 128, ferrous sulfate:
  830, folic acid: 272

Fero-Grad 500 Filmtabs (M)
  ascorbic acid: 128,
  ferrous sulfate: 830

Fero-Gradumet: 830
  (ferrous sulfate)

Fer-Regules (M)
  dioctyl sodium sulfosuccinate: 832,
  ferrous fumarate: 830

ferrocholinate: 830
  (Chel-Iron, Ferrolip)

Ferrolip: 830
  (ferrocholinate)

Ferro-Sequels (M)
  dioctyl sodium sulfosuccinate: 832,
  ferrous fumarate: 830

ferrous fumarate: 830
  (Feostat, Ircon, Toleron)

ferrous gluconate: 830
  (Fergon)

ferrous sulfate: 830
  (Feosol, Fer-in-Sol, Fero-Gradumet,
  Mol-Iron)

Festalan Tabs (M)
  atropine: 132

Fiogesic (M)
  aspirin: 112, pheniramine:
  756, D, pyrilamine: 756, D,
  phenylpropanolamine: 444

Fiorinal (M)
  aspirin: 112, butalbital: 772, D,
  caffeine: 146, phenacetin: 432

Fiorinal with Codeine (M)
  aspirin: 112, butalbital: 772, D,
  caffeine: 146, codeine: 192, D,
  phenacetin: 432

5-FU: 764
  (fluorouracil)

Flagyl: 384
  (metronidazole)

flavoxate: 738
  (Urispas)

Flaxedil: 802
  (gallamine)

Fleet Theophylline: 902, F-12
  (theophylline)

Flexeril: 868, D
  (cyclobenzaprine)

Florinef: 266
  (fludrocortisone)

floxuridine: 764
  (FUDR)

flucytosine: 838
  (Ancobon)

fludrocortisone: 266
  (Florinef)

flumethiazide: 882, F-8

flunitrazepam: 268, D

Fluoromar: 270, D
  (fluroxene)

fluorouracil: 764
  (Adrucil, Efudex, 5-FU)

Fluothane: 292, D
  (halothane)

fluoxymesterone: 712
  (Halotestin, Ora-Testryl)

fluphenazine: 848, D
  (Permitil, Prolixin)

fluprednisolone: 798
  (Alphadrol)

Gynorest: 860
(dydrogesterone)

halazepam: 774, D
(Paxipam)

Haldol: 290, D
(haloperidol)

Haldrone: 798
(paramethasone)

Haley's M-O (M)
magnesium hydroxide: 334

haloperidol: 290, D
(Haldol)

Halotestin: 712
(fluoxymesterone)

halothane: 292, D
(Fluothane)

Harmonyl: 864, D, F-3
(deserpidine)

Hedulin: 744, F-2
(phenindione)

heparin: 294
(Hepathrom, Heprinar, Lipo-Hepin,
Liquaemin, Panheprin)

Hepathrom: 294
(heparin)

Heprinar: 294
(heparin)

Herplex: 838
(idoxuridine)

hetacillin: 846, F-5
(Versapen, Versapen-K)

Hexa-Betalin: 482
(pyridoxine, vitamin B₆)

Hexadrol: 798
(dexamethasone)

hexafluorenium: 800
(Mylaxen)

Hexavibex: 482
(pyridoxine, vitamin B₆)

hexobarbital: 588, D
(Sombulex)

hexocyclium: 738
(Tral)

hexylcaine: 718
(Cyclaine)

hippuric acid: 892

Hiprex: 360, F-11
(methenamine)

Hispril: 756, D
(diphenylpyraline)

Histadyl: 756, D
(methapyrilene, thenylpyramine)

Histaspan: 756, D
(chlorpheniramine)

Histaspan-D (M)
chlorpheniramine: 756, D,
methscopolamine: 374,
phenylephrine: 442

Histaspan-Plus (M)
chlorpheniramine: 756,
phenylephrine: 442

Hold: 212
(dextromethorphan)

homatropine: 738
(Ru-Spas #2, Sed-Tens SE)

H.P. Acthar Gel: 200
(corticotropin)

Hybephen Elixir, Tabs (M)
atropine: 132, hyoscine: 492, D,
hyoscyamine: 136,
phenobarbital: 434, D

Hycodan (M)
homatropine: 738,
hydrocodone: 840, D

Hycotuss Expectorant (M)
hydrocodone: 840, D

Hydergine (M)
ergot alkaloids: 812

hydralazine: 296, F-8
(Apresoline, Dralzine)

Hydrea: 764
(hydroxyurea)

Hydrex: 882, F-8
(benzthiazide)

hydriodic acid: 828

hydrochlorothiazide: 882, F-8
(Esidrix, HydroDIURIL, Oretic)

hydrocodone: 840, D
(Codone, Dicodid)

hydrocortisone: 202
(A-HydroCort, Cort-Dome, Cortef,
Hydrocortone, Solu-Cortef)

Hydrocortone: 202
(cortisol, hydrocortisone)

HydroDIURIL: 882, F-8
(hydrochlorothiazide)

hydroflumethiazide: 882, F-8
(Diucardin, Saluron)

Hydrolose: 832
(methylcellulose)

hydromorphone: 840, D
(Dilaudid)

Hydromox: 882, F-8
(quinethazone)

Hydromox-R (M)
quinethazone: 882, F-8,
reserpine: 864, D, F-3

Hydropres (M)
hydrochlorothiazide: 882, F-8,
reserpine: 864, D, F-3

Hydroserp (M)
hydrochlorothiazide: 882, F-8,
reserpine: 864, D, F-3

Hydrotensin (M)
hydrochlorothiazide: 882, F-8,
reserpine: 864, D, F-3

hydroxyprogesterone: 860
(Delalutin)

hydroxyurea: 764
(Hydrea)

hydroxyzine: 298, D
(Atarax, Vistaril)

Hygroton: 882, F-8
(chlorthalidone)

hyoscine: 492, D
(Transderm-V)

hyoscyamine: 136
(Anaspaz, Cystospaz, Levsin,
Levsinex)

Hyperstat: 218, F-3
(diazoxide)

ibuprofen: 300
(Motrin, Rufen)

idoxuridine: 838
(Dendrid, Herplex, Stoxil)

Iletin: 304
(insulin)

Ilosone: 252, F-5
(erythromycin estolate)

Ilotycin: 814, F-5
(erythromycin)

Imavate: 888, D
(imipramine)

imipramine: 888, D
(Imavate, Janimine, Presamine,
Tofranil)

Imodium: 752, D
(loperamide)

Imuran: 134
(azathioprine)

Inapsine: 242, D
(droperidol)

Inderal: 476, F-8
(propranolol)

Inderide (M)
hydrochlorothiazide: 882, F-8,
propranolol: 476, F-8

Indocin: 302
(indomethacin)

indomethacin: 302
(Indocin)

influenza vaccine: 608

INH: 310, F-4
(isoniazid)

Inhiston: 756, D
(pheniramine)

Innovar (M)
droperidol: 242, D,
fentanyl: 264, D

insulin: 304
(Iletin)

intramuscular injections: 306

Intropin: 234
(dopamine)

Inversine: 342, F-3
(mecamylamine)

iodinated glycerol: 828
(Organidin)

Ionamin: 770
(phentermine)

Iophed Syrup (M)
calcium iodide: 828, chloral
hydrate: 790, D, ephedrine: 248

ipecac: 308

Ircon: 830
(ferrous fumarate)

iron bile salts: 830
(Bilron)

iron-polysaccharide complex: 830
(Niferex)

iron preparations: 830
(many trade names)

Ismelin: 820, F-3
(guanethidine)

isocarboxazid: 836, F-6
(Marplan)

Isoclor (M)
chlorpheniramine: 756, D,
pseudoephedrine: 596

Isoclor Expectorant (M)
chlorpheniramine: 756, D, codeine:
192, D, pseudoephedrine: 596

isoetharine: 604
(Bronkometer, Bronkosol)

isoflurane: 716, D
(Forane)

isoniazid: 310, F-4
(INH, Nydrazid, Triniad, Uniad)

Isopacin (M)
isoniazid: 310, F-4,
para-aminosalicylic acid: 118

isopropamide iodide: 312
(Darbid)

isoproterenol: 314
(Isuprel)

Isoptin: 910
(verapamil)

Isordil: 316
(isosorbide dinitrate)

Isordil with Phenobarbital (M)
isosorbide dinitrate: 316,
phenobarbital: 434, D

isosorbide dinitrate: 316
(Isordil, Sorbitrate)

isoxsuprine: 896
(Vasodilan)

Isuprel: 314
(isoproterenol)

Isuprel Compound Elixir (M)
ephedrine: 248, isoproterenol:
314, phenobarbital: 434, D,
potassium iodide: 828,
theophylline: 902, F-12

Ivadantin: 400, F-1
(nitrofurantoin)

Janimine: 888, D
(imipramine)

Kafocin: 788
(cephaloglycin)

kanamycin: 704
(Kantrex, Klebcil)

Kantrex: 704
(kanamycin)

Kaochlor: 856, F-13
(potassium chloride)

Kaochlor S-F Liquid: 856, F-13
(potassium chloride)

kaolin: 702

Kaon: 856, F-13
(potassium gluconate)

Kaon-Cl: 856, F-13
(potassium chloride)

Kaopectate (M)
kaolin: 702, pectin: 702

Kaopectate Concentrate (M)
kaolin: 702, pectin: 702

Kappadione: 898
(menadiol sodium, vitamin K₄)

Kato: 856, F-13
(potassium chloride)

Kay Ciel Elixir, Powder: 856, F-13
(potassium chloride)

Kayexalate: 506
(sodium polystyrene
sulfonate resin)

Keflex: 788
(cephalexin)

Keflin: 162
(cephalothin)

Librium: 168, D
  (chlordiazepoxide)

licorice (M)
  carbenoxolone: 154, F-3, F-8

lidocaine: 322, D
  (Xylocaine)

Lidone: 768, D
  (molindone)

Limbitrol (M)
  amitriptyline 888, D,
  chlordiazepoxide: 168, D

Lincocin: 324, F-5
  (lincomycin)

lincomycin: 324, F-5
  (Lincocin)

Lioresal: 868, D
  (baclofen)

liothyronine: 886, F-15
  (Cytomel)

liotrix: 886, F-15
  (Euthroid, Thyrolar)

Lipo-Hepin: 294
  (heparin)

Lipo-Lutin: 860
  (progesterone)

Liquaemin: 294
  (heparin)

Liquamar: 742, F-2
  (phenprocoumon)

Lithane: 326, F-10
  (lithium)

lithium: 326, F-10
  (Eskalith, Lithane, Lithonate,
  Lithotabs)

Lithonate: 326, F-10
  (lithium)

Lithotabs: 326, F-10
  (lithium)

Loestrin (M)
  ethinyl estradiol: 816,
  norethindrone: 404

Lofene (M)
  atropine: 132,
  diphenoxylate: 228, D

Lomotil (M)
  atropine: 132,
  diphenoxylate: 228, D

lomustine: 764
  (CeeNU)

Loniten: 388, F-3
  (minoxidil)

Lo/Ovral (M)
  ethinyl estradiol: 816,
  norgestrel: 576

loperamide: 752, D
  (Imodium)

Lopressor: 382, F-8
  (metoprolol)

Lopurin: 110
  (allopurinol)

lorazepam: 774, D
  (Ativan)

Loridine: 160
  (cephaloridine)

Lotusate: 772, D
  (talbutal)

low-salt milk: 328

loxapine: 330, D
  (Daxolin, Loxitane)

Loxitane: 330, D
  (loxapine)

Ludiomil: 888, D
  (maprotiline)

Lufyllin: 902, F-12
  (dyphylline)

Lufyllin-GG (M)
  dyphylline: 902, F-12

Lugol's Solution: 828
  (strong iodine solution)

Luminal: 434, D
  (phenobarbital)

Lynoral: 816
  (ethinyl estradiol)

Lysodren: 764
  (mitotane)

Maalox (M)
  aluminum hydroxide: 722,
  magnesium hydroxide: 334

Macrodantin: 400, F-1
  (nitrofurantoin)

mafenide: 872
  (Sulfamylon Cream)

Magaldrate (M)
aluminum hydroxide: **722,**
magnesium hydroxide: **334**

Magan: 866
(magnesium salicylate)

Magnatril (M)
aluminum hydroxide gel: **722,**
magnesium hydroxide: **334,**
magnesium trisilicate: **728**

magnesium carbonate: 332

magnesium citrate: 834

magnesium hydroxide: 334
(Milk of Magnesia, Mint-O-Mag)

magnesium oxide: 336
(Par-Mag)

magnesium salicylate: 866
(Durasal, Magan, Mobidin)

magnesium sulfate—oral: 834
(Epsom salts)

**magnesium sulfate—
parenteral: 338, D**

magnesium trisilicate: 728

Mal-O-Fem (M)
estradiol: **816,** testosterone: **712**

Maltsupex: 832
(barley malt extract)

Mandelamine: 360, F-11
(methenamine)

Mandol: 618
(cefamandole)

Mannex: 730
(mannitol hexanitrate)

mannitol: 340
(Osmitrol)

mannitol hexanitrate: 730
(Mannex, Vascunitol)

**Mannitol Hexanitrate with
Phenobarbital (M)**
mannitol hexanitrate: **730,**
phenobarbital: **434, D**

Maolate: 170, D
(chlorphenesin)

maprotiline: 888, D
(Ludiomil)

**Marax DF Syrup,
Marax Tabs (M)**
ephedrine: **248,** hydroxyzine:
298, D, theophylline: **902, F-12**

Marezine: 756, D
(cyclizine)

Marplan: 836, F-6
(isocarboxazid)

Matulane: 464, F-6
(procarbazine)

Maxibolin: 708
(ethylestrenol)

mazindol: 770
(Sanorex)

M-Caps: 362
(methionine)

Measurin: 112
(aspirin)

Mebaral: 772, D
(mephobarbital)

mecamylamine: 342, F-3
(Inversine)

mechlorethamine: 764
(Mustargen)

meclizine: 756, D
(Antivert, Bonine)

meclofenamate: 762
(Meclomen)

Meclomen: 762
(meclofenamate)

Mediatric (M)
conjugated estrogens: **816,** ferrous
sulfate: **830,** methamphetamine:
706, methyltestosterone: **712,**
nicotinamide: **398**

Mediatric Liquid (M)
conjugated estrogens: **816,**
methamphetamine: **706,**
methyltestosterone: **712**

Medrol: 798
(methylprednisolone)

medroxyprogesterone: 586
(Amen, Curretab, Depo-Provera,
P-Medrate-P.A., Provera)

mefenamic acid: 344
(Ponstel)

Mefoxin: 788
(cefoxitin)

methenamine: 360, F-11
(Hiprex, Mandelamine)

Methenamine and Sodium Biphosphate (M)
methenamine: 360, F-11,
sodium acid phosphate: 498

Methergine: 812
(methylergonovine)

methicillin: 844
(Azapen, Celbenin, Staphcillin)

methimazole: 600
(Tapazole)

methionine: 362
(Pedameth, Uracid)

methixene: 738
(Trest)

methocarbamol: 364, D
(Delaxin, Robaxin)

methohexital: 366, D
(Brevital)

Methorate: 212
(dextromethorphan)

Methosarb: 712
(calusterone)

methotrexate: 368
(Mexate)

methotrimeprazine: 370, D
(Levoprome)

methoxamine: 876
(Vasoxyl)

methoxyflurane: 372, D
(Penthrane)

methoxyphenamine: 594
(Orthoxine)

methscopolamine: 374
(Pamine, Scoline)

methsuximide: 870, D
(Celontin)

methyclothiazide: 882, F-8
(Aquatensen, Enduron)

methylcellulose: 832
(Hydrolose)

methyldopa: 376, D, F-3
(Aldomet)

methylergonovine: 812
(Methergine)

methylphenidate: 378
(Ritalin)

methylprednisolone: 798
(Medrol)

methyltestosterone: 712
(Metandren, Oreton-Methyl)

methyprylon: 784, D
(Noludar)

methysergide: 812
(Sansert)

Meticortelone: 798
(prednisolone)

Meticorten: 798
(prednisone)

metoclopramide: 380, D
(Reglan)

metocurine: 802
(Metubine)

metolazone: 882, F-8
(Diulo, Zaroxolyn)

metoprolol: 382, F-8
(Lopressor)

metronidazole: 384
(Flagyl)

Metubine: 802
(metocurine)

Mexate: 368
(methotrexate)

Micrainin (M)
aspirin: 112,
meprobamate: 348, D

Micronor: 404
(norethindrone)

Midamor: 614
(amiloride)

Migral (M)
caffeine: 146, cyclizine: 756, D,
ergotamine: 812

Migralam (M)
caffeine: 146, ergotamine: 812,
phenacetin: 432, pyrilamine:
756, D, salicylamide: 866

Milk of Magnesia: 334
(magnesium hydroxide)

Milontin: 870, D
(phensuximide)

Milpath (M)
meprobamate: 348, D,
tridihexethyl: 738

Milprem (M)
conjugated estrogens: 816,
meprobamate: 348, D

Miltown: 348, D
(meprobamate)

Miltrate (M)
meprobamate: 348, D,
pentaerythritol tetranitrate: 730

mineral oil: 832
(Agoral Plain, Petrogalar)

Minipress: 452, F-3
(prazosin)

Minocin: 386, F-16
(minocycline)

minocycline: 386, F-16
(Minocin)

minoxidil: 388, F-3
(Loniten)

Mintezol: 822
(thiabendazole)

Mint-O-Mag: 334
(magnesium hydroxide)

Miocel (M)
physostigmine: 792

Miochol: 792
(acetylcholine chloride)

Miradon: 744, F-2
(anisindione)

Mithracin: 764
(mithramycin)

mithramycin: 764
(Mithracin)

mitomycin: 764
(Mutamycin)

mitotane: 764
(Lysodren)

Moban: 768, D
(molindone)

Mobidin: 866
(magnesium salicylate)

Moderil: 864, D, F-3
(rescinnamine)

Modicon (M)
ethinyl estradiol: 816,
norethindrone: 404

Mogadon: 774, D
(nitrazepam)

molindone: 768, D
(Lidone, Moban)

Mol-Iron: 830
(ferrous sulfate)

morphine: 390, D

Motrin: 300
(ibuprofen)

moxalactam: 590
(Moxam)

Moxam: 590
(moxalactam)

Mudrane (M)
aminophylline: 902, F-12,
ephedrine: 248, phenobarbital:
434, D, potassium iodide: 828

Mudrane GG Elixir (M)
ephedrine: 248, phenobarbital:
434, D, theophylline: 902, F-12

Mudrane GG Tabs (M)
aminophylline: 902, F-12,
ephedrine: 248, phenobarbital:
434, D

Mustargen: 764
(mechlorethamine)

Mutamycin: 764
(mitomycin)

Mychel: 166
(chloramphenicol)

Mycifradin: 396
(neomycin)

Mylanta (M)
aluminum hydroxide: 722,
magnesium hydroxide: 334

Mylaxen: 800
(hexafluorenium)

Myleran: 144
(busulfan)

Myochrysine: 818
(gold sodium thiomalate)

Myotonachol: 580
(bethanechol)

Mysoline: 456, D
(primidone)

Mysteclin-F (M)
amphotericin B: 120,
tetracycline: 880, F-16

nicotinyl alcohol: 896
(Roniacol)

Nidar (M)
butabarbital: 772, D,
pentobarbital: 430, D,
phenobarbital: 434, D,
secobarbital: 494, D

nifedipine: 910
(Procardia)

Niferex: 830 ·
(iron-polysaccharide complex)

Nipride: 504, F-3
(sodium nitroprusside)

Nisentil: 840, D
(alphaprodine)

nitrazepam: 774, D
(Mogadon)

Nitro-Bid: 402
(nitroglycerin)

nitrofurantoin: 400, F-1
(Cyantin, Furadantin, Ivadantin,
Macrodantin)

nitroglycerin: 402
(Nitro-Bid, Nitroglyn, Nitrol,
Nitrong, Nitrospan, Nitrostat)

Nitroglyn: 402
(nitroglycerin)

Nitrol: 402
(nitroglycerin)

Nitrong: 402
(nitroglycerin)

Nitrospan: 402
(nitroglycerin)

Nitrostat: 402
(nitroglycerin)

nitrous oxide: 716, D

Noctec: 790, D
(chloral hydrate)

No Doz: 146
(caffeine)

Nolamine (M)
chlorpheniramine: 756, D,
phenindamine: 756, D,
phenylpropanolamine: 444

Noludar: 784, D
(methyprylon)

Nolvadex: 764
(tamoxifen)

norepinephrine: 318
(Levophed)

norethandrolone: 708

norethindrone: 404
(Micronor, Norlutate, Norlutin,
Nor-Q.D.)

norethynodrel: 860

Norflex: 408, D
(orphenadrine)

Norgesic, Norgesic Forte (M)
aspirin: 112, caffeine: 146,
orphenadrine: 408, D,
phenacetin: 432

norgestrel: 576
(Ovrette)

Norinyl (M)
mestranol: 816,
norethindrone: 404

**Norisodrine Syrup with
Calcium Iodide (M)**
calcium iodide: 828,
isoproterenol: 314

Norlestrin (M)
ethinyl estradiol: 816,
norethindrone: 404

Norlutate: 404
(norethindrone)

Norlutin: 404
(norethindrone)

Norpace: 230
(disopyramide)

Norpramin: 888, D
(desipramine)

Nor-Q.D.: 404
(norethindrone)

nortriptyline: 888, D
(Aventyl, Pamelor)

Nospaz: 220
(dicyclomine)

Novafed: 596
(pseudoephedrine)

Novafed A (M)
chlorpheniramine: 756, D,
pseudoephedrine: 596

Novahistine DH (M)
chlorpheniramine: 756, D,
codeine: 192, D,
phenylpropanolamine: 444

Novahistine DMX (M)
dextromethorphan: 212,
pseudoephedrine: 596

Novahistine Elixir, Tablets (M)
chlorpheniramine: 756, D,
phenylpropanolamine: 444

Novahistine Expectorant (M)
codeine: 192, D,
phenylpropanolamine: 444

Novahistine LP (M)
chlorpheniramine: 756, D,
phenylephrine: 442

Novocain: 462
(procaine)

NTZ Solution (M)
phenylephrine: 442,
thenyldiamine: 756, D

Nubain: 840, D
(nalbuphine)

Nucofed (M)
codeine: 192, D,
pseudoephedrine: 596

Numorphan: 840, D
(oxymorphone)

Nupercainal: 718
(dibucaine)

Nupercaine: 718
(dibucaine)

Nutrajel: 722
(aluminum hydroxide)

Nydrazid: 310, F-4
(isoniazid)

nylidrin: 896
(Arlidin)

Obetrol (M)
amphetamine: 706,
dextroamphetamine: 706,
methamphetamine: 706

Obotan: 706
(dextroamphetamine)

Ogen: 816
(estrone)

Omnipen: 122, F-5
(ampicillin—oral)

Omnipen-N: 122
(ampicillin—injection)

Omni-Tuss (M)
chlorpheniramine: 756, D,
codeine: 192, D,
ephedrine: 248,
phenyltoloxamine: 756, D

Oncovin: 562
(vincristine)

opium alkaloids: 406, D
(Pantopon)

opium tincture: 752, D

**opium tincture,
camphorated:** 752, D
(Paregoric)

Optimine: 756, D
(azatadine)

Oracon (M)
dimethisterone: 860,
ethinyl estradiol: 816

Ora-Testryl: 712
(fluoxymesterone)

Oratrol: 782, D
(dichlorphenamide)

Orazinc: 570
(zinc sulfate)

Oretic: 882, F-8
(hydrochlorothiazide)

Oreticyl, Oreticyl Forte (M)
deserpidine: 864, D, F-3,
hydrochlorothiazide: 882, F-8

Oreton: 712
(testosterone)

Oreton-Methyl: 712
(methyltestosterone)

Organidin: 828
(iodinated glycerol)

Orinase: 544
(tolbutamide)

Ornade (M)
chlorpheniramine: 756, D,
isopropamide: 312,
phenylpropanolamine: 444

Ornex (M)
acetaminophen: 102,
phenylpropanolamine: 444

orphenadrine: 408, D
(Disipal, Norflex)

Ortho-Novum (M)
mestranol: 816,
norethindrone: 404

Orthoxine: 594
(methoxyphenamine)

Osmitrol: 340
(mannitol)

Otobione (M)
cortisol: **202,** neomycin: **396,**
polymyxin B sulfate: **450**

Otrivin: 876
(xylometazoline)

Ovcon (M)
ethinyl estradiol: **816,**
norethindrone: **404**

Ovral (M)
ethinyl estradiol: **816,**
norgestrel: **576**

Ovrette: 576
(norgestrel)

Ovulen (M)
ethynodiol diacetate: **860,**
mestranol: **816**

oxacillin—injection: 410
(Bactocill, Prostaphlin)

oxacillin—oral: 410, F-5
(Bactocill, Prostaphlin)

Oxaine (M)
aluminum hydroxide gel: **722**

Oxaine-M (M)
aluminum hydroxide gel: **722,**
magnesium hydroxide: **334**

Oxalid: 414
(oxyphenbutazone)

oxandrolone: 708
(Anavar)

oxazepam: 774, D
(Serax)

oxtriphylline: 902, F-12
(Choledyl)

oxybutynin: 738
(Ditropan)

oxycodone: 412, D

Oxy-Kesso-Tetra: 416, F-16
(oxytetracycline)

oxymetazoline: 876
(Afrin)

oxymetholone: 708
(Adroyd, Anadrol)

oxymorphone: 840, D
(Numorphan)

oxyphenbutazone: 414
(Oxalid, Tandearil)

oxyphencyclimine: 738
(Daricon)

oxyphenonium: 738
(Antrenyl)

oxytetracycline: 416, F-16
(Dalimycin, Oxy-Kesso-Tetra,
Terramycin)

PABA: 116
(Pabagel, Pabanol, PreSun,
Ray-Nox, Sunbrella)

Pabagel: 116
(aminobenzoic acid, PABA,
para-aminobenzoic acid)

Pabalate (M)
para-aminobenzoic acid: **116,**
sodium salicylate: **866**

Pabanol: 116
(aminobenzoic acid, PABA,
para-aminobenzoic acid)

Pagitane: 736, D
(cycrimine)

Pamelor: 888, D
(nortriptyline)

Pamine: 374
(methscopolamine)

pancuronium: 802
(Pavulon)

Panheprin: 294
(heparin)

Panmycin: 880, F-16
(tetracycline)

Pantopon: 406, D
(opium alkaloids)

Panwarfin: 568, F-2
(warfarin)

**Papavatral,
Papavatral L.A. (M)**
ethaverine: **896,**
pentaerythritol tetranitrate: **730**

papaverine: 418
(Cerespan, Pavabid, Pavacap,
Paverine, P-200, Therapav,
Vasospan)

para-aminobenzoic acid: 116
(Pabagel, Pabanol, PreSun,
Ray-Nox, Sunbrella)

penicillin G benzathine—
oral: 846, F-5
(Bicillin)

penicillin G potassium—
injection: 422
(Pfizerpen)

penicillin G potassium—
oral: 422, F-5
(G-Recillin-T, Pentids, Pfizerpen G,
SK-Penicillin G, Sugracillin)

penicillin G procaine: 844
(Crysticillin A.S., Duracillin A.S.,
Pfizerpen AS, Tu-Cillin, Wycillin)

penicillin V: 846, F-5
(Compocillin V, V-Cillin)

penicillin V benzathine: 844

penicillin V
potassium: 424, F-5
(Betapen-VK, Compocillin-VK,
Ledercillin VK, Penapar VK,
Penicillin VK, Pen-Vee K,
Pfizerpen VK, Robicillin VK,
SK-Penicillin VK, Uticillin VK,
V-Cillin K, Veetids)

Penicillin VK: 424, F-5
(penicillin V potassium)

Pennpheno (M)
pentaerythritol tetranitrate: 730,
phenobarbital: 434, D

Pensyn: 122, F-5
(ampicillin—oral)

pentaerythritol tetranitrate: 730
(Duotrate, Pentritol, Peritrate)

pentazocine: 428, D
(Talwin)

Penthrane: 372, D
(methoxyflurane)

Pentids: 422, F-5
(penicillin G potassium—oral)

pentobarbital: 430, D
(Nembutal)

pentolinium: 760, F-3
(Ansolysen)

Pentothal: 532, D
(thiopental)

Pentritol: 730
(pentaerythritol tetranitrate)

pentylenetetrazol: 786

Pen-Vee K: 424, F-5
(penicillin V potassium)

Pepto-Bismol: 866
(bismuth subsalicylate)

Pep-Aid: 146
(caffeine)

Percocet-5 (M)
acetaminophen: 102,
oxycodone: 412, D

Percodan (M)
aspirin: 112, oxycodone: 412, D

Percogesic (M)
acetaminophen: 102,
phenyltoloxamine: 756, D

Percogesic-C (M)
acetaminophen: 102, codeine:
192, D, phenyltoloxamine: 756, D

Percorten: 210
(desoxycorticosterone)

Periactin: 756, D
(cyproheptadine)

Peritrate: 730
(pentaerythritol tetranitrate)

Peritrate with
Nitroglycerin (M)
nitroglycerin: 402,
pentaerythritol tetranitrate: 730

Peritrate with
Phenobarbital (M)
pentaerythritol tetranitrate: 730,
phenobarbital: 434, D

Permapen: 844
(penicillin G benzathine—injection)

Permitil: 848, D
(fluphenazine)

perphenazine: 848, D
(Trilafon)

Persantine: 730
(dipyridamole)

Pertofrane: 888, D
(desipramine)

Petrogalar: 832
(mineral oil)

Pfizer-E: 814, F-5
(erythromycin)

Pfizerpen: 422
(penicillin G potassium—injection)

Pfizerpen-AS: 844
(penicillin G procaine)

Pfizerpen G: 422, F-5
(penicillin G potassium—oral)

Pfizerpen VK: 424, F-5
(penicillin V potassium)

Phazyme PB Tabs (M)
phenobarbital: 434, D

phenacemide: 746, D
(Phenurone)

phenacetin: 432

Phenaphen: 102
(acetaminophen)

Phenaphen with Codeine (M)
acetaminophen: 102,
codeine: 192, D

phenazopyridine: 822
(Pyridium)

phendimetrazine: 770
(Bacarate, Plegine, Statobex)

phenelzine: 836, F-6
(Nardil)

Phenergan: 758, D
(promethazine)

Phenergan Compound (M)
aspirin: 112, promethazine:
758, D, pseudoephedrine: 596

Phenergan-D (M)
promethazine: 758, D,
pseudoephedrine: 596

Phenergan Expectorant (M)
promethazine: 758, D

**Phenergan Expectorant with
Codeine (M)**
codeine: 192, D,
promethazine: 758, D

Phenergan Pediatric (M)
dextromethorphan: 212,
promethazine: 758, D

**Phenergan VC Expectorant
with Codeine (M)**
codeine: 192, D, phenylephrine:
442, promethazine: 758, D

phenindamine: 756, D

phenindione: 744, F-2
(Hedulin)

pheniramine: 756, D
(Inhiston)

phenmetrazine: 770
(Preludin)

phenobarbital: 434, D
(Eskabarb, Luminal, Sedadrops)

phenolphthalein: 832
(Alophen, Ex-Lax, Feen-A-Mint)

Phenoxene: 172, D
(chlorphenoxamine)

phenoxybenzamine: 436, F-3
(Dibenzyline)

phenprocoumon: 742, F-2
(Liquamar)

phensuximide: 870, D
(Milontin)

phentermine: 770
(Adipex-8, Adipex-P, Fastin,
Ionamin, Tora)

phentolamine: 438, F-3
(Regitine)

Phenurone: 746, D
(phenacemide)

phenylbutazone: 440
(Azolid, Butazolidin)

phenylephrine: 442
(Alconefrin, Neo-Synephrine)

phenylpropanolamine: 444
(Propadrine)

phenyl salicylate: 866

phenyltoloxamine: 756, D

Phenylzin Drops (M)
phenylephrine: 442

phenytoin: 446, D, F-1
(Dilantin)

pHos-pHaid (M)
ammonium acid phosphate: 892,
sodium acid phosphate: 498,
sodium acid pyrophosphate: 892

Phosphaljel: 722
(aluminum phosphate)

Phospholine Iodide: 244
(echothiophate)

Phospho-Soda: 498
(sodium acid phosphate, sodium
biphosphate)

physostigmine: 792
(Antilirium)

Rautrax (M)
flumethiazide: 882, F-8,
potassium chloride: 856, F-13,
rauwolfia serpentina: 864, D, F-3

Rautrax-N (M)
bendroflumethiazide: 882, F-8,
potassium chloride: 856, F-13,
rauwolfia serpentina: 864, D, F-3

Rautrax-N Modified (M)
bendroflumethiazide: 882, F-8,
rauwolfia serpentina: 864, D, F-3

Rauwiloid: 864, D, F-3
(alseroxylon)

rauwolfia serpentina: 864, D, F-3
(Raudixin)

Rauzide (M)
bendroflumethiazide: 882, F-8,
rauwolfia serpentina: 864, D, F-3

Ray-Nox: 116
(aminobenzoic acid, PABA,
para-aminobenzoic acid)

Regitine: 438, F-3
(phentolamine)

Reglan: 380, D
(metoclopramide)

Regonol: 792
(pyridostigmine)

Regroton (M)
chlorthalidone: 882, F-8,
reserpine: 864, D, F-3

Rela: 156, D
(carisoprodol)

Remsed: 758, D
(promethazine)

Renese: 882, F-8
(polythiazide)

Renese-R (M)
polythiazide: 882, F-8,
reserpine: 864, D, F-3

Renoquid: 872
(sulfacytine)

Repoise: 848, D
(butaperazine)

rescinnamine: 864, D, F-3
(Moderil)

reserpine: 864, D, F-3
(Reserpoid, Sandril, Serpasil)

Reserpoid: 864, D, F-3
(reserpine)

Restoril: 774, D
(temazepam)

Rhinex D-Lay (M)
acetaminophen: 102,
chlorpheniramine: 756, D,
phenylpropanolamine: 444,
salicylamide: 866

Rifadin: 490, F-5
(rifampin)

Rifamate (M)
isoniazid: 310, F-4,
rifampin: 490, F-5

rifampin: 490, F-5
(Rifadin, Rimactane)

Rimactane: 490, F-5
(rifampin)

Riopan, Riopan Plus (M)
aluminum hydroxide: 722,
magnesium hydroxide: 334

Ritalin: 378
(methylphenidate)

Robalate: 722
(dihydroxyaluminum aminoacetate)

Robamox: 846, F-5
(amoxicillin)

Robam-Petn (M)
meprobamate: 348, D,
pentaerythritol tetranitrate: 730

Robaxin: 364, D
(methocarbamol)

Robaxisal (M)
aspirin: 112,
methocarbamol: 364, D

Robenecol (M)
probenecid: 458

Robicillin VK: 424, F-5
(penicillin V potassium)

Ro-Bile Tabs (M)
belladonna: 136

Robimycin: 814, F-5
(erythromycin)

Robinul: 284, D
(glycopyrrolate)

**Robinul-PH,
Robinul-PH Forte (M)**
glycopyrrolate: 284, D,
phenobarbital: 434, D

Robitet: 880, F-16
(tetracycline)

Robitussin A-C (M)
codeine: 192, D

Robitussin-CF (M)
dextromethorphan: 212,
phenylpropanolamine: 444

Robitussin-DAC (M)
codeine: 192, D,
pseudoephedrine: 596

Robitussin-DM (M)
dextromethorphan: 212

Robitussin-PE (M)
pseudoephedrine: 596

Rolaids: 722
(dihydroxyaluminum
sodium carbonate)

**Rondec C, Rondec D Oral
Drops, Rondec S,
Rondec T (M)**
carbinoxamine: 756, D,
pseudoephedrine: 596

Rondec DM Drops, Syrup (M)
carbinoxamine: 756, D,
dextromethorphan: 212,
pseudoephedrine: 596

Rondomycin: 880, F-16
(methacycline)

Roniacol: 896
(nicotinyl alcohol)

RP-Mycin: 814, F-5
(erythromycin)

Rufen: 300
(ibuprofen)

Ru-Spas #2: 738
(homatropine)

Rynatan (M)
chlorpheniramine: 756, D,
phenylephrine: 442,
pyrilamine: 756, D

Rynatuss (M)
carbetapentane: 736, D,
chlorpheniramine: 756, D,
ephedrine: 248,
phenylephrine: 442

Salcoce (M)
sodium salicylate: 866

Sal Hepatica (M)
sodium acid phosphate: 498,
sodium bicarbonate: 500, F-17

salicylamide: 866
(Amid-Sal, Salrin)

Salrin: 866
(salicylamide)

salsalate: 866
(Arcylate, Disalcid)

salt: 502
(sodium chloride)

**salt substitutes containing
potassium: 854**

Saluron: 882, F-8
(hydroflumethiazide)

Salutensin (M)
hydroflumethiazide: 882, F-8,
reserpine: 864, D, F-3

Sandoptal: 772, D
(butalbital)

Sandril: 864, D, F-3
(reserpine)

Sanorex: 770
(mazindol)

Sansert: 812
(methysergide)

S.A.S.-500: 522
(sulfasalazine)

Savacort-50, Savacort-100: 798
(prednisolone)

Savacort-S (M)
prednisolone: 798

S.B.P. (M)
butabarbital: 772, D,
phenobarbital: 434, D,
secobarbital: 494, D

S.B.P. Plus (M)
butabarbital: 772, D,
homatropine: 738,
phenobarbital: 434, D,
secobarbital: 494, D

Scoline: 374
(methscopolamine)

scopolamine: 492, D
(Transderm-V)

secobarbital: 494, D
(Seconal)

Seconal: 494, D
(secobarbital)

Sedadrops: 434, D
(phenobarbital)

Suladyne (M)
phenazopyridine: 822, sulfadiazine: 872, sulfamethizole: 514

Sulcolon: 522
(sulfasalazine)

sulfabenzamide: 872

sulfacetamide: 872

sulfacytine: 872
(Renoquid)

sulfadiazine: 872

sulfamerazine: 872

sulfameter: 872
(Sulla)

sulfamethazine: 872

sulfamethizole: 514
(Thiosulfil)

sulfamethoxazole: 516
(Gantanol)

Sulfamylon Cream: 872
(mafenide)

sulfanilamide: 872

sulfapyridine: 872

sulfasalazine: 522
(Azulfidine, S.A.S.-500, Sulcolon)

sulfathiazole: 872

sulfinpyrazone: 524
(Anturane)

sulfisoxazole: 526
(Gantrisin, SK-Soxazole)

sulfoxone: 838
(Diasone)

sulindac: 606
(Clinoril)

Sulla: 872
(sulfameter)

Sumox: 846, F-5
(amoxicillin)

Sumycin: 880, F-16
(tetracycline)

Sunbrella: 116
(aminobenzoic acid, PABA, para-aminobenzoic acid)

suramin: 838
(Antrypol, Bayer-205)

Surfacaine: 718
(cyclomethycaine)

Surital: 530, D
(thiamylal)

Surmontil: 888, D
(trimipramine)

Sus-Phrine: 250
(epinephrine)

Sustaire: 902, F-12
(theophylline)

Sux-Cert: 512
(succinylcholine)

Symmetrel: 114
(amantadine)

Synalgos (M)
aspirin: 112, caffeine: 146, phenacetin: 432, promethazine: 758, D

Synalgos-DC (M)
aspirin: 112, caffeine: 146, dihydrocodeine: 192, D, phenacetin: 432, promethazine: 758, D

Syncurine: 800
(decamethonium)

Synkayvite: 898
(menadiol sodium, vitamin K₄)

Synthroid: 886, F-15
(levothyroxine)

syrosingopine: 864, D, F-3
(Singoserp)

Tacaryl: 758, D
(methdilazine)

TACE: 816
(chlorotrianisene)

Tagamet: 180
(cimetidine)

talbutal: 772, D
(Lotusate)

Talwin: 428, D
(pentazocine)

Talwin Compound (M)
aspirin: 112, pentazocine: 428, D

tamoxifen: 764
(Nolvadex)

Tandearil: 414
(oxyphenbutazone)

TAO: 556
(troleandomycin)

Tral: 738
(hexocyclium)

Trancopal: 780, D
(chlormezanone)

Transderm-V: 492, D
(hyoscine, scopolamine)

Tranxene: 774, D
(clorazepate)

tranylcypromine: 836, F-6
(Parnate)

Trecator-SC: 822
(ethionamide)

Tremin: 550, D
(trihexyphenidyl)

Trest: 738
(methixene)

Trialka Liquid (M)
aluminum hydroxide: 722,
magnesium hydroxide: 334

Trialka Tablets: 726, F-17
(calcium carbonate)

triamcinolone: 798
(Aristocort, Kenacort)

Triaminic (M)
pheniramine: 756, D,
phenylpropanolamine: 444,
pyrilamine: 756, D

Triaminic Decongestant Cough Syrup (M)
ammonium chloride: 892,
dextromethorphan: 212,
pheniramine: 756, D,
phenylpropanolamine: 444,
pyrilamine: 756, D

Triaminic Expectorant DH (M)
hydrocodone: 840, D,
pheniramine: 756, D,
phenylpropanolamine: 444,
pyrilamine: 756, D

Triaminic Expectorant with Codeine (M)
codeine: 192, D,
phenylpropanolamine: 444

triamterene: 546, F-3
(Dyrenium)

Triavil (M)
amitriptyline: 888, D,
perphenazine: 848, D

trichlormethiazide: 882, F-8
(Metahydrin, Naqua)

triclofos: 548, D
(Triclos)

Triclos: 548, D
(triclofos)

tridihexethyl: 738
(Pathilon)

Tridione: 552, D
(trimethadione)

trifluoperazine: 848, D
(Stelazine)

triflupromazine: 848, D
(Vesprin)

trihexyphenidyl: 550, D
(Artane, Tremin)

Trilafon: 848, D
(perphenazine)

Trilisate (M)
choline salicylate: 866,
magnesium salicylate: 866

trimeprazine: 758, D
(Temaril)

trimethadione: 552, D
(Tridione)

trimethaphan: 760, F-3
(Arfonad)

trimethobenzamide: 554
(Tigan)

trimipramine: 888, D
(Surmontil)

Trimox: 846, F-5
(amoxicillin)

Trind (M)
acetaminophen: 102,
phenylephrine: 442

Trind-DM (M)
acetaminophen: 102,
dextromethorphan: 212,
phenylephrine: 442

Triniad: 310, F-4
(isoniazid)

Triniad Plus 30 (M)
isoniazid: 310, F-4,
pyridoxine: 482

tripelennamine: 756, D
(PBZ)

Triple Barbiturate Elixir (M)
butabarbital: **772, D,**
pentobarbital: **430, D,**
phenobarbital: **434, D**

Triple Sulfa (M)
sulfadiazine: **872,** sulfamerazine:
872, sulfamethazine: **872**

triprolidine: 756, D
(Actidil)

Trisogel (M)
aluminum hydroxide: **722,**
magnesium trisilicate: **728**

trisulfapyrimidines (M)
sulfadiazine: **872,** sulfamerazine:
872, sulfamethazine: **872**

Triten: 756, D
(dimethindene)

Trocinate: 738
(thiphenamil)

troleandomycin: 556
(TAO)

tubocurarine: 802

Tu-Cillin: 844
(penicillin G procaine)

Tuinal (M)
amobarbital: **772, D,**
secobarbital: **494, D**

Tums: 726, F-17
(calcium carbonate)

Tussade: 212
(dextromethorphan)

Tussagesic (M)
acetaminophen: **102,**
dextromethorphan: **212,**
pheniramine: **756, D,**
phenylpropanolamine: **444,**
pyrilamine: **756, D**

Tussar SF, Tussar-2 Syrup (M)
carbetapentane: **736, D,**
chlorpheniramine: **756, D,**
codeine: **192, D**

**Tussend Expectorant, Liquid,
Tabs (M)**
hydrocodone: **840, D,**
pseudoephedrine: **596**

Tussionex (M)
hydrocodone: **840, D,**
phenyltoloxamine: **756, D**

**Tussi-Organidin DM
Elixir (M)**
chlorpheniramine: **756, D,**
dextromethorphan: **212,**
iodinated glycerol: **828**

Tussi-Organidin Elixir (M)
chlorpheniramine: **756, D,**
codeine: **192, D,**
iodinated glycerol: **828**

Tuss-Ornade (M)
caramiphen: **736, D,**
chlorpheniramine: **756, D,**
isopropamide: **312,**
phenylpropanolamine: **444**

tybamate: 780, D
(Tybatran)

Tybatran: 780, D
(tybamate)

Tylenol: 102
(acetaminophen)

Tylenol with Codeine (M)
acetaminophen: **102,**
codeine: **192, D**

Tylox (M)
acetaminophen: **102,**
oxycodone: **412, D**

tyramine-containing foods: 890

Tyzine: 876
(tetrahydrozoline)

Ultracef: 788
(cefadroxil)

Uniad: 310, F-4
(isoniazid)

Uniad-Plus (M)
isoniazid: **310, F-4,**
pyridoxine: **482**

Unipen (injection): 844
(nafcillin—injection)

Unipen (oral): 846, F-5
(nafcillin—oral)

Unipres (M)
hydralazine: **296, F-8,**
hydrochlorothiazide: **882, F-8,**
reserpine: **864, D, F-3**

Unitensen: 760, F-3
(cryptenamine)

Uracel: 866
(sodium salicylate)

Uracid: 362
(methionine)

uracil mustard: 764

Urecholine: 580
(bethanechol)

Urised (M)
atropine: **132,** hyoscyamine: **136,**
methenamine: **360, F-11,**
phenyl salicylate: **866**

Urispas: 738
(flavoxate)

Urobiotic (M)
oxytetracycline: **416, F-16,**
phenazopyridine: **822,**
sulfamethizole: **514**

Uro-K: 892
(potassium acid phosphate)

Uro-Phosphate (M)
methenamine: **360, F-11,**
sodium acid phosphate: **498**

Uroqid-Acid (M)
methenamine: **360, F-11,**
sodium acid phosphate: **498**

Uticillin VK: 424, F-5
(penicillin V potassium)

Uticort: 798
(betamethasone)

Utimox: 846, F-5
(amoxicillin)

vaccine, BCG: 822

vaccine, influenza: 608

vaccines, live (smallpox et al): 496

Vagitrol (M)
sulfanilamide: **872**

Valisone: 798
(betamethasone)

Valium: 216, D, F-1
(diazepam)

Vallestril: 816
(methallenestril)

Valmid: 258, D
(ethinamate)

Valpin: 738
(anisotropine)

Valpin 50-PB Tabs (M)
anisotropine: **738,**
phenobarbital: **434, D**

valproic acid: 558, D
(Depakene)

Vanceril: 798
(beclomethasone)

Vancocin: 560
(vancomycin)

vancomycin: 560
(Vancocin)

Van-Mox: 846, F-5
(amoxicillin)

Vanquish (M)
acetaminophen: **102,** aluminum
hydroxide gel: **722,** aspirin: **112,**
caffeine: **146,**
magnesium hydroxide: **334**

Vaponefrin: 250
(epinephrine)

Vaporole: 730
(amyl nitrite)

Vascunitol: 730
(mannitol hexanitrate)

Vasocon-A (M)
naphazoline: **876**

Vasodilan: 896
(isoxsuprine)

Vasospan: 418
(papaverine)

Vasoxyl: 876
(methoxamine)

V-Cillin: 846, F-5
(penicillin V)

V-Cillin K: 424, F-5
(penicillin V potassium)

Veetids: 424, F-5
(penicillin V potassium)

Velban: 764
(vinblastine)

Velosef: 164
(cephradine)

Ventaire: 480
(protokylol)

Ventolin: 876
(albuterol)

Veracillin: 846, F-5
(dicloxacillin)

SECTION II
Number Index

HOW TO USE THIS SECTION

The NUMBER INDEX is STEP 2 in locating an interaction description (see "How to Use This Book," page v). Consult this section to find the *interaction number(s)* for your drugs of interest.

For example: You want to know if drug #384 interacts with drug #568. Here's what to do:

Find the 384 group of numbers in this section, and scan the list for 568; or find the 568 group, and scan for 384. In either case, the *interaction number* for that drug pair, I-299, will follow:

384-108: **I-133**	*OR*	568-288: **I-293**
-140: **I-299**		-302: **I-295**
-166: **I-459**		-344: **I-297**
-232: **I-555**		-366: **I-267**
-568: **I-299**		-384: **I-299**

(Each interaction has been assigned an arbitrary, odd-numbered code.)

When the number pair you're looking for does not appear in this section, it means that our current research has not uncovered any significant, adverse interaction between the two drugs involved.

This section can also be used to find *every* interaction listed for any *one* given drug. Just find the group of numbers for the drug in question, where you'll see numbers listed for all the drugs it reacts with, along with corresponding interaction numbers. (To convert drug numbers into generic names, use the APPENDIX.)

Once you've found the interaction number or numbers of interest, proceed to Section III: INTERACTIONS (gray-edged pages).

176-104: I-339
-108: I-115
-110: I-149
-112: I-667
-138: I-351
-166: I-455
-186: I-473
-202: I-337
-214: I-353
-234: I-351
-248: I-351
-250: I-351
-254: I-339
-274: I-347
-276: I-339
-280: I-341
-304: I-655
-314: I-351
-318: I-351
-350: I-339
-354: I-351
-378: I-351
-382: I-335
-392: I-335
-414: I-659
-440: I-659
-442: I-351
-444: I-351
-446: I-345
-458: I-665
-464: I-347
-476: I-335
-480: I-351
-490: I-227
-514: I-669
-516: I-669
-522: I-669
-526: I-669
-592: I-351
-594: I-351
-596: I-351
-598: I-351
-602: I-351
-604: I-351
-706: I-351
-708: I-193
-776: I-335
-782: I-339
-798: I-337
-820: I-343
-824: I-345
-836: I-347
-866: I-667
-872: I-669
-876: I-351
-878: I-351
-882: I-339
-886: I-353
-890: I-351
178-140: I-275
-214: I-465
-222: I-463
-224: I-463
-568: I-275
-742: I-275
-744: I-275
-804: I-463
-886: I-465
180-140: I-261
-146: I-727
-168: I-695
-188: I-695
-216: I-695
-268: I-695
-332: I-699
-334: I-699
-336: I-699
-382: I-405
-390: I-685
-392: I-405
-406: I-685
-412: I-685
-446: I-649
-476: I-405
-500: I-699
-568: I-261
-620: I-743
-722: I-699
-726: I-699
-728: I-699
-742: I-261
-752: I-685
-774: I-695
-776: I-405
-824: I-649
-840: I-685
-902: I-663
182-166: I-459
-278: I-171
-396: I-171
-496: I-371
-510: I-171
-538: I-171
-704: I-171
184-166: I-451
-192: I-355
-228: I-355
-252: I-471
-270: I-199
-292: I-199
-372: I-199
-512: I-469
-702: I-103
-716: I-199
-752: I-355
-800: I-469
-802: I-469
-814: I-471
186-140: I-277
-176: I-473
-544: I-473
-568: I-277
-742: I-277
-744: I-277
-826: I-473
188-166: I-459
-174: I-329
-180: I-695
-260: I-329
-290: I-329
-320: I-403
-330: I-329
-352: I-629
-370: I-329
-404: I-325
-466: I-329
-468: I-329
-472: I-329
-490: I-697
-576: I-325
-584: I-325
-586: I-325
-758: I-329
-768: I-329
-816: I-325
-848: I-329
-860: I-325
-884: I-329

-412: I-741	-862: I-233	-722: I-735	-438: I-231
-416: I-615	-876: I-539	-726: I-735	-446: I-701
-428: I-741	-878: I-539	-728: I-735	-452: I-231
-442: I-539	-880: I-615	-736: I-241	-470: I-255
-444: I-539	-882: I-537	-738: I-243	-476: I-231
-470: I-741	-890: I-539	-756: I-235	-490: I-701
-474: I-741	-910: I-201	-758: I-235	-492: I-239
-480: I-539	226-114: I-239	-768: I-235	-504: I-231
-492: I-741	-118: I-181	-848: I-235	-508: I-231
-498: I-537	-132: I-243	-862: I-239	-546: I-231
-508: I-547	-136: I-243	-884: I-235	-550: I-239
-512: I-509	-166: I-459	-888: I-235	-616: I-231
-522: I-549	-172: I-241	228-184: I-355	-736: I-239
-550: I-741	-174: I-235	-224: I-741	-738: I-255
-592: I-539	-220: I-243	-324: I-357	-760: I-231
-594: I-539	-224: I-741	230-132: I-255	-776: I-231
-596: I-539	-230: I-239	-136: I-255	-820: I-231
-598: I-539	-260: I-241	-172: I-239	-824: I-701
-602: I-539	-284: I-241	-190: I-231	-864: I-231
-604: I-539	-290: I-235	-218: I-231	-882: I-231
-702: I-105	-298: I-235	-220: I-255	-888: I-573
-706: I-539	-312: I-243	-226: I-239	232-108: I-123
-722: I-213	-320: I-237	-254: I-231	-140: I-283
-726: I-213	-330: I-235	-260: I-239	-310: I-553
-728: I-213	-332: I-735	-276: I-231	-352: I-629
-736: I-741	-334: I-735	-284: I-239	-384: I-555
-738: I-741	-336: I-735	-296: I-231	-420: I-557
-752: I-741	-370: I-235	-312: I-255	-446: I-551
-778: I-425	-374: I-243	-342: I-231	-568: I-283
-782: I-537	-408: I-241	-350: I-231	-742: I-283
-798: I-537	-466: I-235	-374: I-255	-744: I-283
-800: I-509	-468: I-235	-376: I-231	-824: I-551
-802: I-509	-470: I-243	-382: I-231	234-138: I-439
-814: I-615	-472: I-235	-388: I-231	-146: I-439
-832: I-537	-492: I-241	-392: I-231	-176: I-351
-834: I-537	-500: I-735	-408: I-239	-190: I-367
-840: I-741	-550: I-241	-436: I-231	-218: I-367

-836: **I-439**
-864: **I-367**
-876: **I-439**
-878: **I-439**
-882: **I-367**
-888: **I-135**
-890: **I-439**
-902: **I-439**
356-150: **I-577**
-224: **I-741**
-366: **I-577**
-430: **I-577**
-434: **I-577**
-446: **I-577**
-456: **I-577**
-490: **I-577**
-494: **I-577**
-530: **I-577**
-532: **I-577**
-588: **I-577**
-772: **I-577**
-824: **I-577**
360-104: **I-563**
-332: **I-563**
-334: **I-563**
-336: **I-563**
-500: **I-563**
-514: **I-569**
-516: **I-569**
-522: **I-569**
-526: **I-569**
-722: **I-563**
-726: **I-563**
-728: **I-563**
-782: **I-563**
-872: **I-569**
362-320: **I-661**

364-108: **I-119**
366-108: **I-117**
-140: **I-267**
-166: **I-459**
-174: **I-329**
-202: **I-385**
-210: **I-385**
-222: **I-387**
-240: **I-389**
-260: **I-329**
-266: **I-385**
-272: **I-391**
-288: **I-393**
-290: **I-329**
-330: **I-329**
-352: **I-629**
-356: **I-577**
-370: **I-329**
-382: **I-381**
-392: **I-381**
-404: **I-325**
-446: **I-395**
-466: **I-329**
-468: **I-329**
-472: **I-329**
-476: **I-381**
-490: **I-399**
-568: **I-267**
-576: **I-325**
-584: **I-325**
-586: **I-325**
-742: **I-267**
-744: **I-267**
-758: **I-329**
-768: **I-329**
-776: **I-381**
-798: **I-385**

-816: **I-325**
-824: **I-395**
-848: **I-329**
-860: **I-325**
-862: **I-397**
-884: **I-329**
-888: **I-333**
-902: **I-349**
368-112: **I-457**
-166: **I-459**
-352: **I-629**
-440: **I-545**
-458: **I-431**
-496: **I-371**
-514: **I-163**
-516: **I-163**
-522: **I-163**
-526: **I-163**
-866: **I-457**
-872: **I-163**
370-104: **I-329**
-132: **I-255**
-136: **I-255**
-138: **I-187**
-146: **I-373**
-150: **I-329**
-166: **I-459**
-168: **I-329**
-172: **I-235**
-188: **I-329**
-190: **I-361**
-216: **I-329**
-218: **I-361**
-220: **I-255**
-224: **I-741**
-226: **I-235**
-250: **I-571**

-254: **I-361**
-260: **I-235**
-268: **I-329**
-276: **I-361**
-284: **I-235**
-296: **I-361**
-312: **I-255**
-320: **I-359**
-322: **I-329**
-326: **I-593**
-332: **I-221**
-334: **I-221**
-336: **I-221**
-342: **I-361**
-350: **I-361**
-366: **I-329**
-374: **I-255**
-376: **I-361**
-382: **I-361**
-388: **I-361**
-392: **I-361**
-408: **I-235**
-420: **I-329**
-430: **I-329**
-434: **I-329**
-436: **I-361**
-438: **I-361**
-446: **I-329**
-452: **I-361**
-456: **I-329**
-470: **I-255**
-476: **I-361**
-492: **I-235**
-494: **I-329**
-504: **I-361**
-508: **I-361**
-530: **I-329**

-772: **I-381**
-800: **I-409**
-802: **I-409**
-826: **I-335**
-836: **I-417**
-848: **I-361**
-862: **I-231**
-866: **I-415**
-876: **I-367**
-878: **I-367**
-884: **I-361**
-888: **I-155**
-890: **I-367**
-896: **I-229**
-902: **I-383**
-910: **I-619**
394 -140: **I-301**
-568: **I-301**
-742: **I-301**
-744: **I-301**
396 -120: **I-159**
-148: **I-165**
-152: **I-167**
-160: **I-169**
-162: **I-169**
-164: **I-169**
-182: **I-171**
-196: **I-175**
-198: **I-175**
-224: **I-543**
-270: **I-161**
-278: **I-157**
-292: **I-161**
-372: **I-161**
-404: **I-107**
-450: **I-175**
-510: **I-157**

-512: **I-173**
-536: **I-167**
-538: **I-157**
-560: **I-177**
-564: **I-179**
-576: **I-107**
-584: **I-107**
-586: **I-107**
-590: **I-169**
-618: **I-169**
-704: **I-157**
-716: **I-161**
-788: **I-169**
-800: **I-173**
-802: **I-173**
-816: **I-107**
-860: **I-107**
398 -352: **I-629**
400 -166: **I-459**
-352: **I-629**
-404: **I-107**
-458: **I-411**
-524: **I-413**
-576: **I-107**
-584: **I-107**
-586: **I-107**
-728: **I-737**
-816: **I-107**
-860: **I-107**
402 -108: **I-111**
-190: **I-231**
-218: **I-231**
-254: **I-231**
-276: **I-231**
-296: **I-231**
-342: **I-231**
-350: **I-231**

-376: **I-231**
-382: **I-231**
-388: **I-231**
-392: **I-231**
-418: **I-229**
-436: **I-231**
-438: **I-231**
-452: **I-231**
-476: **I-231**
-504: **I-231**
-508: **I-231**
-542: **I-229**
-546: **I-231**
-616: **I-231**
-760: **I-231**
-776: **I-231**
-820: **I-231**
-864: **I-231**
-882: **I-231**
-896: **I-229**
404 -104: **I-325**
-122: **I-107**
-128: **I-609**
-140: **I-279**
-146: **I-375**
-150: **I-325**
-166: **I-107**
-168: **I-325**
-188: **I-325**
-202: **I-489**
-210: **I-489**
-216: **I-325**
-240: **I-107**
-266: **I-489**
-268: **I-325**
-272: **I-575**
-322: **I-325**

-352: **I-629**
-366: **I-325**
-386: **I-107**
-396: **I-107**
-400: **I-107**
-416: **I-107**
-420: **I-325**
-424: **I-107**
-430: **I-325**
-434: **I-325**
-446: **I-325**
-456: **I-325**
-482: **I-585**
-490: **I-107**
-494: **I-325**
-514: **I-107**
-516: **I-107**
-522: **I-107**
-526: **I-107**
-530: **I-325**
-532: **I-325**
-552: **I-325**
-556: **I-709**
-558: **I-325**
-588: **I-325**
-742: **I-279**
-744: **I-279**
-746: **I-325**
-772: **I-325**
-774: **I-325**
-798: **I-489**
-824: **I-325**
-846: **I-107**
-870: **I-325**
-872: **I-107**
-880: **I-107**

-470: **I-243**
-472: **I-235**
-500: **I-735**
-550: **I-241**
-722: **I-735**
-726: **I-735**
-728: **I-735**
-736: **I-241**
-738: **I-243**
-756: **I-235**
-758: **I-235**
-768: **I-235**
-848: **I-235**
-862: **I-239**
-884: **I-235**
-888: **I-235**
494-108: **I-117**
-140: **I-267**
-166: **I-459**
-174: **I-329**
-202: **I-385**
-210: **I-385**
-222: **I-387**
-240: **I-389**
-260: **I-329**
-266: **I-385**
-272: **I-391**
-288: **I-393**
-290: **I-329**
-330: **I-329**
-352: **I-629**
-356: **I-577**
-370: **I-329**
-382: **I-381**
-392: **I-381**
-404: **I-325**
-446: **I-395**

-466: **I-329**
-468: **I-329**
-472: **I-329**
-476: **I-381**
-490: **I-399**
-568: **I-267**
-576: **I-325**
-584: **I-325**
-586: **I-325**
-742: **I-267**
-744: **I-267**
-758: **I-329**
-768: **I-329**
-776: **I-381**
-798: **I-385**
-816: **I-325**
-824: **I-395**
-848: **I-329**
-860: **I-325**
-862: **I-397**
-884: **I-329**
-888: **I-333**
-902: **I-349**
496-106: **I-371**
-130: **I-371**
-134: **I-371**
-144: **I-371**
-158: **I-371**
-182: **I-371**
-202: **I-505**
-204: **I-371**
-210: **I-505**
-238: **I-371**
-266: **I-505**
-352: **I-371**
-368: **I-371**
-464: **I-371**

-534: **I-371**
-562: **I-371**
-764: **I-371**
-798: **I-505**
498-200: **I-507**
-202: **I-499**
-210: **I-499**
-222: **I-537**
-224: **I-537**
-266: **I-499**
-512: **I-521**
-798: **I-499**
-800: **I-521**
-802: **I-521**
-804: **I-537**
500-112: **I-205**
-132: **I-735**
-136: **I-735**
-138: **I-189**
-172: **I-735**
-180: **I-699**
-220: **I-735**
-226: **I-735**
-240: **I-217**
-284: **I-735**
-312: **I-735**
-342: **I-137**
-360: **I-563**
-374: **I-735**
-382: **I-211**
-386: **I-217**
-392: **I-211**
-408: **I-735**
-416: **I-217**
-460: **I-717**
-470: **I-735**
-476: **I-211**

-492: **I-735**
-550: **I-735**
-596: **I-639**
-706: **I-189**
-736: **I-735**
-738: **I-735**
-776: **I-211**
-830: **I-215**
-862: **I-247**
-866: **I-205**
-880: **I-217**
502-326: **I-589**
504-132: **I-231**
-138: **I-367**
-174: **I-361**
-230: **I-231**
-234: **I-367**
-246: **I-231**
-248: **I-367**
-250: **I-367**
-260: **I-361**
-274: **I-705**
-290: **I-361**
-314: **I-367**
-316: **I-231**
-318: **I-367**
-322: **I-231**
-330: **I-361**
-354: **I-367**
-370: **I-361**
-378: **I-367**
-402: **I-231**
-442: **I-367**
-444: **I-367**
-460: **I-231**
-464: **I-705**
-466: **I-361**

-234: I-439
-236: I-439
-248: I-439
-250: I-439
-254: I-367
-274: I-439
-276: I-367
-296: I-367
-304: I-351
-314: I-439
-318: I-439
-332: I-639
-334: I-639
-336: I-639
-342: I-367
-350: I-367
-354: I-439
-376: I-367
-378: I-439
-382: I-367
-388: I-367
-392: I-367
-436: I-367
-438: I-367
-442: I-439
-444: I-439
-452: I-367
-464: I-439
-474: I-441
-476: I-367
-480: I-439
-500: I-639
-504: I-367
-508: I-367
-544: I-351
-546: I-367
-592: I-439

-594: I-439
-598: I-439
-602: I-439
-604: I-439
-616: I-367
-706: I-439
-722: I-639
-726: I-639
-728: I-639
-760: I-367
-770: I-439
-776: I-367
-782: I-639
-786: I-439
-804: I-539
-812: I-561
-820: I-367
-826: I-351
-836: I-439
-864: I-367
-876: I-439
-878: I-439
-882: I-367
-890: I-439
-902: I-439
598 -138: I-439
-146: I-439
-176: I-351
-190: I-367
-218: I-367
-222: I-539
-224: I-539
-234: I-439
-236: I-439
-248: I-439
-250: I-439
-254: I-367

-274: I-439
-276: I-367
-296: I-367
-304: I-351
-314: I-439
-318: I-439
-342: I-367
-350: I-367
-354: I-439
-376: I-367
-378: I-439
-382: I-367
-388: I-367
-392: I-367
-436: I-367
-438: I-367
-442: I-439
-444: I-439
-452: I-367
-464: I-439
-474: I-441
-476: I-367
-480: I-439
-504: I-367
-508: I-367
-544: I-351
-546: I-367
-592: I-439
-594: I-439
-596: I-439
-602: I-439
-604: I-439
-616: I-367
-706: I-439
-760: I-367
-770: I-439
-776: I-367

-786: I-439
-804: I-539
-812: I-561
-820: I-367
-826: I-351
-836: I-439
-864: I-367
-876: I-439
-878: I-439
-882: I-367
-888: I-135
-890: I-439
-902: I-439
600 -140: I-307
-294: I-307
-568: I-307
-742: I-307
-744: I-307
602 -138: I-439
-146: I-439
-176: I-351
-190: I-367
-218: I-367
-222: I-539
-224: I-539
-234: I-439
-236: I-439
-248: I-439
-250: I-439
-254: I-367
-274: I-439
-276: I-367
-296: I-367
-304: I-351
-314: I-439
-318: I-439
-342: I-367

-836: **I-705**
-848: **I-361**
-862: **I-231**
-876: **I-367**
-878: **I-367**
-884: **I-361**
-890: **I-367**
762-112: **I-369**
-276: **I-703**
-300: **I-369**
-302: **I-369**
-326: **I-731**
-344: **I-369**
-382: **I-415**
-392: **I-415**
-414: **I-369**
-440: **I-369**
-476: **I-415**
-606: **I-369**
-762: **I-369**
-776: **I-415**
-866: **I-369**
-882: **I-703**
764-166: **I-459**
-496: **I-371**
768-104: **I-329**
-132: **I-255**
-136: **I-255**
-146: **I-373**
-150: **I-329**
-168: **I-329**
-172: **I-235**
-188: **I-329**
-190: **I-361**
-216: **I-329**
-218: **I-361**
-220: **I-255**

-226: **I-235**
-250: **I-571**
-254: **I-361**
-260: **I-235**
-268: **I-329**
-276: **I-361**
-284: **I-235**
-296: **I-361**
-312: **I-255**
-322: **I-329**
-342: **I-361**
-350: **I-361**
-366: **I-329**
-374: **I-255**
-376: **I-361**
-382: **I-361**
-388: **I-361**
-392: **I-361**
-408: **I-235**
-420: **I-329**
-430: **I-329**
-434: **I-329**
-436: **I-361**
-438: **I-361**
-446: **I-329**
-452: **I-361**
-456: **I-329**
-470: **I-255**
-476: **I-361**
-492: **I-235**
-494: **I-329**
-504: **I-361**
-508: **I-361**
-530: **I-329**
-532: **I-329**
-546: **I-361**
-550: **I-235**

-552: **I-329**
-558: **I-329**
-588: **I-329**
-616: **I-361**
-736: **I-235**
-738: **I-255**
-746: **I-329**
-760: **I-361**
-772: **I-329**
-774: **I-329**
-776: **I-361**
-820: **I-491**
-824: **I-329**
-864: **I-361**
-870: **I-329**
-882: **I-361**
770-138: **I-439**
-146: **I-439**
-234: **I-439**
-236: **I-439**
-248: **I-439**
-250: **I-439**
-274: **I-439**
-314: **I-439**
-318: **I-439**
-354: **I-439**
-378: **I-439**
-442: **I-439**
-444: **I-439**
-464: **I-439**
-474: **I-441**
-480: **I-439**
-592: **I-439**
-594: **I-439**
-596: **I-439**
-598: **I-439**
-602: **I-439**

-604: **I-439**
-706: **I-439**
-770: **I-439**
-786: **I-439**
-836: **I-439**
-876: **I-439**
-878: **I-439**
-890: **I-439**
-902: **I-439**
772-108: **I-117**
-140: **I-267**
-166: **I-459**
-174: **I-329**
-202: **I-385**
-210: **I-385**
-222: **I-387**
-240: **I-389**
-260: **I-329**
-266: **I-385**
-272: **I-391**
-288: **I-393**
-290: **I-329**
-330: **I-329**
-352: **I-629**
-356: **I-577**
-370: **I-329**
-382: **I-381**
-392: **I-381**
-404: **I-325**
-446: **I-395**
-466: **I-329**
-468: **I-329**
-472: **I-329**
-476: **I-381**
-490: **I-399**
-568: **I-267**
-576: **I-325**

Interactions

HOW TO USE THIS SECTION

The INTERACTIONS section is STEP 3 in locating an interaction description (see "How to Use This Book," page v). Consult this section after finding the interaction number or numbers (in Section II: NUMBER INDEX) for one or more pairs of drugs.

Interaction numbers are arbitrarily chosen, consecutive odd numbers. Interaction descriptions are listed here in numerical order according to interaction number.

Each interaction description is a concise précis of essential facts, highlighting the information most useful for *actual clinical practice.* Each description is supplemented with suggestions for treating, minimizing, and/or preventing adverse effects.

Since most interaction descriptions involve more than one pair of drugs, you will often find headings that look like this:

ANTIDIABETIC AGENTS	⟷	BETA BLOCKERS
176 544		382 476
304 826		392 776

The numbers displayed under each drug or group name represent *all* the drugs that react as described. To convert the numbers back into drug names, turn to the APPENDIX, which lists generic names by number and provides information on the clinical orientation of each drug or drug class.

The **FOOD INTERACTIONS** section begins on page 260. Drugs that react with foods are listed in the **NAME INDEX** with "F" numbers, corresponding to specific descriptions in the **FOOD INTERACTIONS** section.

Drugs with CNS depressant activity are flagged with a "D" in the **NAME INDEX**. When more than one "D" drug is taken, the depressant effects are additive. Whenever you are dealing with two or more such drugs, see Interaction #I-435.

ACETAMINOPHEN ⟷ ALCOHOL

102   108

Reaction: Patients who regularly consume substantial amounts of alcohol are at increased risk of hepatotoxicity from either acute overdoses or chronic use of large amounts (3.0-8.0 gm/day) of acetaminophen.

Suggestion: Heavy users of alcohol should avoid more than an occasional dose of acetaminophen.

ADSORBENTS ⟷ LINCOMYCIN/
CLINDAMYCIN

702   184   324

Reactions: Oral lincomycin absorption is decreased about 90%; oral clindamycin absorption may be decreased.

Suggestions: Try to avoid this combination. If it cannot be avoided, give the adsorbent more than 3 hours before the lincomycin or clindamycin.

ADSORBENTS ⟷ DIGOXIN

702   224

Reaction: Decreased absorption of digoxin; decreased digoxin effect.

Suggestion: Give digoxin 2 hours before or 2 hours after the adsorbent.

Note: Prolonged diarrhea (for which adsorbents may be used) can cause hypokalemia, increasing the risk of digitalis toxicity (see Interaction #I-537).

I-107

ANTIBIOTICS   ⟷   CONTRACEPTIVES, ORAL/ESTROGENS

122	416	522		404	586
166	424	526		576	816
240	490	846		584	860
386	514	872			
396	516	880			
400					

Reaction: Many antibiotics (ampicillin, chloramphenicol, neomycin, nitrofurantoin, penicillin V, rifampin, sulfonamides, tetracyclines) may increase the hepatic metabolism or decrease the absorption of estrogens, and thus of most oral contraceptives, possibly increasing the risk of pregnancy.

Possible exceptions are contraceptives that contain only progestogens: #404 norethindrone (Micronor, Nor-Q.D.) or #576 norgestrel (Ovrette).

Suggestions: Oral contraceptives may be unreliable during therapy with any of the antibiotics with numbers listed above. Patients should abstain from intercourse or use alternative methods of contraception. Breakthrough bleeding should be considered evidence of a reaction.

Patients taking estrogens for other purposes may require dosage adjustments.

I-109

THEOPHYLLINE AND OTHER XANTHINES   ⟷   TROLEANDOMYCIN

902   556

Reaction: Up to 50% increase in serum theophylline levels (via inhibition of theophylline metabolism), possibly leading to toxicity. Toxic effects may include GI upset with nausea and vomiting, headache, irritability, dizziness, tremors, insomnia, seizures, tachycardia, cardiac arrhythmias.

Suggestions: In patients with therapeutic serum theophylline levels, reduce theophylline dosage by 50% when starting troleandomycin. Measure serum theophylline levels after 3 to 4 days of combined therapy, and adjust dosage accordingly.

Advise patients to promptly report any toxic symptoms.

Note: These other xanthines may react the same way: #902 aminophylline; #902 oxtriphylline. Dyphylline (#902) is excreted as unchanged drug in the urine and is unlikely to interact.

I-111

ALCOHOL $\longleftrightarrow$ ANTIANGINAL AGENTS

108

316	402	730
382	476	776
392		

Reaction: Additive hypotension. Severity depends on the amount of alcohol consumed. Postural hypotension (dizziness, light-headedness, weakness) may progress to syncope and severe hypotension.

Suggestions: Patients taking antianginal drugs should limit alcohol intake to less than 4 ounces in any 24-hour period.

Advise patients to lie down immediately, rest, then change position slowly if early symptoms of postural hypotension occur.

I-113

ALCOHOL $\longleftrightarrow$ ANTICOAGULANTS, ORAL

108

140	742
568	744

Reactions: 1. Increased anticoagulant effect in acute alcohol intoxication.
2. Decreased anticoagulant effect in chronic alcohol use.

Suggestions: 1. Acute alcohol intoxication substantially prolongs prothrombin time, increasing the risk of hemorrhage, in patients taking anticoagulants. Patients should limit alcohol intake to less than 4 ounces in any 24-hour period. Should acute intoxication occur, wait 1 to 2 days before giving the next anticoagulant dose.
2. Regular, non-acute alcohol use may increase anticoagulant dosage requirements. Monitor prothrombin time frequently in patients who drink, and adjust anticoagulant dosage accordingly.

I-115

ALCOHOL   ⟷   ANTIDIABETIC AGENTS

108

176   544
304   826

Reactions: 1. Unpredictable and varying alterations in blood sugar—most serious is severe hypoglycemia.
2. Possible disulfiram-like reaction: dyspnea, dizziness, facial flushing, severe headache.

Suggestions: 1. Patients taking antidiabetic drugs should limit alcohol intake to less than 4 ounces in any 24-hour period.

Measure urine and blood sugar levels frequently in patients who drink acutely or chronically, and adjust dosage of antidiabetic agent accordingly.

Advise patients to promptly report any symptoms of hypoglycemia: faintness, weakness, sweating, palpitations, tachycardia, headache, confusion, ataxia, visual disturbances. Also advise patients to keep a candy bar, sugar cube, or other source of simple carbohydrate readily available for emergencies.
2. Patients who have had a disulfiram-like reaction should avoid all alcohol, including alcohol-containing medications. Exposure to alcohol-based paints or cosmetics may also cause a reaction in susceptible individuals.

Notes: The disulfiram-like reaction is most likely to occur with chlorpropamide.

In some patients, 325 mg of aspirin given 1 hour before alcohol consumption may prevent the disulfiram-like reaction.

ALCOHOL   ⟷   BARBITURATES/
PRIMIDONE

108

366	456	532
430	494	588
434	530	772

Reactions: **1.** Decreased barbiturate effect in chronic alcohol
use.
       2. Additive CNS depression with acute alcohol
intoxication.

Suggestions: **1.** Patients taking barbiturates should limit alcohol
intake to less than 4 ounces in any 24-hour period.
If larger quantities of alcohol are regularly
consumed, barbiturate metabolism may be
increased.
       2. Warn patients that acute alcohol intoxication
produces additive impairment of driving ability in
combination with barbiturates. (See Interaction
#I-435).

Note: Primidone (#456) is metabolized to phenobarbital and will
cause the same reactions.

ALCOHOL   ⟷   CARBAMATES

108

156	348	582
170	364	780
258		

Reactions: **1.** Additive CNS depression in acute alcohol
intoxication.
       2. Decreased carbamate effect in chronic alcohol use.

Suggestions: **1.** Warn patients that alcohol and carbamates have
additive effects in impairing driving ability. (See
Interaction #I-435.)
       2. Patients taking carbamates should avoid regular
alcohol use, as well as acute intoxication.

I-121

ALCOHOL   ⟷   CHLORAL DERIVATIVES/ TRICLOFOS

108   548   790

Reactions: 1. Disulfiram-like reaction: dyspnea, dizziness, facia! flushing, severe headache.
2. Additive CNS depression.

Suggestions: 1. Patients taking chloral derivatives should avoid all alcohol, including alcohol-containing medications. Exposure to alcohol-based paints or cosmetics may also cause a reaction in susceptible individuals.
2. Warn patients that combining alcohol and chloral hydrate may greatly impair driving ability. (See Interaction #I-435.)

Note: Triclofos (#548) is chemically related to chloral derivatives and can cause the same reactions.

I-123

ALCOHOL   ⟷   DISULFIRAM

108   232

Reaction: "Disulfiram reaction": dyspnea, dizziness, facial flushing, severe headache, chest pain, blurred vision, thirst, nausea, vomiting.

Suggestion: Patients taking disulfiram should avoid all alcohol, including alcohol-containing medications. Exposure to alcohol-based paints or cosmetics may also cause a reaction in susceptible individuals.

I-125

TETRACYCLINES   ⟷   ZINC SULFATE

240   416   570
386   880

Reaction: Decreased absorption of tetracycline (exceptions: #240 doxycycline and probably #386 minocycline).

Suggestion: If these agents must be given together, separate the doses by at least 2 hours.

See Food Interaction #F-16.

ALCOHOL   ⟷   GUANETHIDINE

108   820

Reaction: Additive hypotension. Severity depends principally on the amount of alcohol consumed. Postural hypotension (dizziness, light-headedness, weakness) may progress to syncope.

Suggestions: Patients taking guanethidine should limit alcohol intake to less than 4 ounces in any 24-hour period.

Advise patients to lie down immediately, rest, then change position slowly if early symptoms of postural hypotension occur.

Warn patients that postural hypotension is more likely after prolonged standing, exercise, during hot weather, or when rising suddenly from a lying or sitting position.

ALCOHOL   ⟷   PHENYTOIN AND
                          OTHER HYDANTOINS

108   446   824

Reactions: 1. Additive sedative and anticonvulsant effects in acute alcohol intoxication.
                 2. Decreased anticonvulsant effect in chronic alcohol use.

Suggestions: 1. See Interaction #I-435.
                 2. Monitor chronic alcohol users for decreased anticonvulsant effect, and increase anticonvulsant dosage accordingly.

Note: While this interaction is usually described as Alcohol-Phenytoin, the other hydantoins (#824 ethotoin and #824 mephenytoin) can probably cause the same reactions.

ALCOHOL   ⟷   ISONIAZID

108   310

Reactions: 1. Possible decreased therapeutic response to isoniazid in chronic alcohol use.
                 2. Possible additive hepatotoxicity.

continued

I-131

continued

Suggestions: Heavy users of alcohol may be at increased risk of isoniazid hepatitis and should be monitored for evidence of hepatic dysfunction.

Advise patients to promptly report any of these symptoms: loss of appetite, fatigue, weakness, nausea, vomiting, dark urine, light-colored stools, yellowing of skin or eyes.

I-133

ALCOHOL   ⟷   METRONIDAZOLE

108   384

Reaction: Mild disulfiram-like reaction occurs infrequently. Symptoms include dyspnea, dizziness, facial flushing, severe headache.

Suggestion: Patients taking metronidazole should avoid all alcohol, including alcohol-containing medications. Exposure to alcohol-based paints or cosmetics may also cause a reaction in susceptible individuals.

I-135

SYMPATHOMIMETICS,   ⟷   TRICYCLIC
DIRECT-ACTING   ANTIDEPRESSANTS

234	318	480	602	888
248	354	592	604	
250	442	594	876	
314	444	598	878*	

Reaction: Increased adrenergic effect, possibly resulting in arrhythmias or severe hypertensive crisis with hyperpyrexia, severe headache, visual disturbances, encephalopathy.

Suggestions: Use this combination only with great caution and in a controlled environment.

Patients taking tricyclic antidepressants should seek professional advice before using any nonprescription nose drops or cold remedies, as many contain direct-acting sympathomimetics.

The direct-acting sympathomimetics include:

albuterol
dobutamine
dopamine
ephedrine
epinephrine
ethylnorepinephrine
isoetharine
isoproterenol
levarterenol
mephentermine
metaproterenol
metaraminol

methoxamine
methoxyphenamine
naphazoline
norepinephrine
oxymetazoline
phenylephrine
phenylpropanolamine
propylhexedrine
protokylol
terbutaline
tetrahydrozoline
xylometazoline

Note: Local anesthetic preparations often contain epinephrine (eg, Xylocaine with Epinephrine).

*Mephentermine (#878) is both direct- and indirect-acting. Other drugs in the #878 group do not participate in this interaction.

MECAMYLAMINE   ⟷   URINARY ALKALINIZERS

342

104	336	726
332	500	728
334	722	782

Reaction: Alkalinization of the urine increases the reabsorption of mecamylamine; excessive hypotension can result.

Suggestions: Patients taking mecamylamine should try to avoid urinary alkalinizers. Antacid use should be limited, and sodium bicarbonate should be avoided. Excessive amounts of alkalinizing foods (dairy products, vegetables, citrus juices, nuts) should also be avoided.

Advise patients to sit or lie down quickly if dizziness or light-headedness occurs.

I-139

ALCOHOL   ⟷   RIFAMPIN

108   490

Reactions: **1.** Possible decreased rifampin effect.
             2. Possible additive hepatotoxicity.

Suggestions: Patients taking rifampin should avoid regular alcohol use and acute intoxication. Occasional alcohol use should be limited to less than 4 ounces in any 24-hour period.

Heavy drinkers may be at increased risk of hepatitis and should be monitored for evidence of hepatic dysfunction.

Advise patients to promptly report any of these symptoms: loss of appetite, fatigue, weakness, nausea, vomiting, dark urine, light-colored stools, yellowing of skin or eyes.

I-141

ALCOHOL   ⟷   SALICYLATES

108   112   866

Reaction: Additive gastric irritation and increased risk of occult or frank GI bleeding.

Suggestions: Patients taking salicylates should avoid alcohol, especially if there is a past history of peptic ulcer, gastric irritation or bleeding.

Chronic alcohol users may be at less risk of GI bleeding when taking magnesium salicylate, sodium salicylate, choline salicylate, salsalate, or salicylamide instead of aspirin.

Advise patients on long-term salicylate therapy to promptly report any unusual weakness, gastric distress, black or tarry stools.

Note: Pepto-Bismol (bismuth subsalicylate) is an unexpected source of significant amounts of salicylate.

ALLOPURINOL   ⟷   ANTICOAGULANTS, ORAL

110

140   742
568   744

Reaction: Possible increased anticoagulant effect.

Suggestion: Monitor prothrombin time, and adjust anticoagulant dosage, if needed, when starting or stopping allopurinol.

ALLOPURINOL   ⟷   AZATHIOPRINE

110   134

Reaction: Azathioprine is rapidly metabolized to mercaptopurine. Allopurinol decreases mercaptopurine metabolism, leading to increased blood levels and possible toxicity. Toxic effects may include nausea and vomiting, liver damage (with possible jaundice and itching), bone marrow depression (with chills, fever, sore throat, mouth sores, unusual bruising or bleeding, unusual tiredness or weakness).

Suggestions: If concurrent therapy is needed, reduce azathioprine to $\frac{1}{3}$ or $\frac{1}{4}$ of usual dosage, and monitor mercaptopurine blood levels.

Advise patients to promptly report any toxic symptoms.

ALLOPURINOL   ⟷   CYCLOPHOSPHAMIDE

110   204

Reaction: Increase in cyclophosphamide levels, possibly leading to toxicity. Toxic effects may include nausea and vomiting, alopecia, hemorrhagic cystitis, bone marrow depression (with chills, fever, sore throat, mouth sores, unusual bruising or bleeding, unusual tiredness or weakness).

Suggestions: When concurrent allopurinol therapy is unavoidable, monitor patients frequently for evidence of cyclophosphamide toxicity.

Advise patients to promptly report any toxic symptoms.

I-149

ALLOPURINOL   ⟷   HYPOGLYCEMICS, ORAL

110   176   544   826

Reaction: Possible increased hypoglycemic effect (documented only with chlorpropamide, to date). Symptoms of hypoglycemia may include faintness, weakness, sweating, palpitations, tachycardia, headache, confusion, ataxia, visual disturbances.

Suggestions: Monitor urine and blood sugar frequently, and adjust hypoglycemic dosage as needed, when adding or stopping allopurinol.

If control proves difficult, insulin can be substituted for the oral hypoglycemic.

Advise patients to promptly report any symptoms of hypoglycemia. Also advise patients to keep a candy bar, sugar cube, or other source of simple carbohydrate readily available for emergencies.

I-151

ALLOPURINOL   ⟷   MERCAPTOPURINE

110   352

Reactions: Increase in mercaptopurine blood levels, possibly leading to toxicity. Toxic effects may include nausea and vomiting, liver damage (with possible jaundice and itching), bone marrow depression (with chills, fever, sore throat, mouth sores, unusual bruising or bleeding, unusual tiredness or weakness). Additive liver damage may also occur.

Suggestions: If concurrent allopurinol therapy is unavoidable, reduce mercaptopurine to $\frac{1}{3}$ or $\frac{1}{4}$ of usual dosage, and periodically monitor mercaptopurine blood levels and liver function.

Advise patients to promptly report any toxic symptoms.

I-153

ALLOPURINOL   ⟷   PROBENECID

110   458

Reaction: Possible decreased metabolism of probenecid. This may increase the risk of precipitation of urates or urate precursors in the kidneys.

Suggestions: When this combination is required, patients should increase fluid intake to 2–3 quarts per day. Consider alkalinization of the urine in patients at high risk of urate nephrolithiasis.

I-155

BETA BLOCKERS   ⟷   TRICYCLIC ANTIDEPRESSANTS

382	476	888
392	776	

Reaction: Decreased beta blocker effect.

Suggestion: If response to beta blocker is inadequate, the tricyclic antidepressant could be the cause. Adjust dosages or change agents accordingly.

I-157

AMINOGLYCOSIDES   ⟷   AMINOGLYCOSIDES

(Every drug with number listed below interacts with every other drug in the list.)

278   510   704
396   538

Reaction: Severe additive ototoxicity and nephrotoxicity. Ototoxic effects are frequently permanent.

Suggestions: Avoid concurrent or sequential use of more than one aminoglycoside, either topically or systemically.

Monitor patients for evidence of ototoxicity (dizziness, vertigo, tinnitus, nausea, vomiting, hearing loss) and nephrotoxicity (hematuria, oliguria, polydipsia, anorexia, nausea, vomiting, weakness, drowsiness, dizziness, dyspnea).

I-159

AMINOGLYCOSIDES   ⟷   AMPHOTERICIN B

278   510   704   120
396   538

Reaction: Additive nephrotoxicity.

Suggestions: If this combination is unavoidable, monitor renal function (BUN and urine specific gravity) frequently.

I-159
continued

Monitor patients for evidence of nephrotoxicity: hematuria, oliguria, polydipsia, anorexia, nausea, vomiting, weakness, drowsiness, dizziness, dyspnea.

I-161

AMINOGLYCOSIDES ⟷ GENERAL ANESTHETICS, INHALATION

278	510	704		270	372
396	538			292	716

Reaction: Aminoglycosides increase neuromuscular blockade caused by general inhalation anesthetics; respiratory depression progressing to apnea can result. This reaction is most frequent with #396 neomycin.

Suggestions: When inhalation anesthesia follows aminoglycoside therapy, observe patients closely for evidence of respiratory depression.

Neostigmine reverses the neuromuscular blockade.

I-163

METHOTREXATE ⟷ SULFONAMIDES

368		514	522	872
		516	526	

Reaction: Increase in serum methotrexate levels, possibly leading to toxicity. Toxic effects may include nausea, vomiting, diarrhea, skin and mouth ulcers, GI bleeding, alopecia, skin rashes, renal and hepatic damage, bone marrow depression leading to septicemia.

Suggestions: Try to avoid this combination; toxic reaction may be severe.

If concurrent use is unavoidable, monitor serum methotrexate levels, and adjust dosage accordingly. Advise patients to promptly report any toxic symptoms.

AMINOGLYCOSIDES ⟷ CAPREOMYCIN

278 510 704   148
396 538

Reaction: Nephrotoxic and ototoxic effects of aminoglycosides may be enhanced. Nephrotoxic effects may include hematuria, oliguria, polydipsia, anorexia, nausea, vomiting, weakness, drowsiness, dizziness, dyspnea. Ototoxic effects may include dizziness, vertigo, tinnitus, nausea, vomiting, hearing loss.

Suggestion: This combination is usually avoidable.

AMINOGLYCOSIDES ⟷ CARBENICILLIN/
                   TICARCILLIN

278 510 704   152 536
396 538

Reactions: Inactivation of aminoglycoside (especially gentamicin or tobramycin) when mixed with carbenicillin or ticarcillin in the same IV solution. Inactivation can also occur in patients with severe renal failure, even when the drugs are given separately. Amikacin reacts less than other aminoglycosides.

Suggestions: Do not mix these drugs in IV solution. If they must be given IV, administer them 2 hours apart in separate IV infusions.

In cases of severe renal failure, reduce carbenicillin or ticarcillin dosage accordingly, and monitor serum aminoglycoside levels.

AMINOGLYCOSIDES ⟷ CEPHALOSPORINS

278 510 704   160 164 618
396 538   162 590 788

Reaction: Possible additive nephrotoxicity.

Suggestion: Monitor renal function, and watch for evidence of nephrotoxicity: hematuria, oliguria, polydipsia, anorexia, nausea, vomiting, weakness, drowsiness, dizziness, dyspnea.

I-171

AMINOGLYCOSIDES ⟷ CISPLATIN

278 510 704   182
396 538

Reaction: Possible additive ototoxicity and nephrotoxicity. Ototoxic effects can be severe and permanent.

Suggestions: When this combination is unavoidable, monitor patients for evidence of ototoxicity (dizziness, vertigo, tinnitus, nausea, vomiting, hearing loss) and nephrotoxicity (hematuria, oliguria, polydipsia, anorexia, nausea, vomiting, weakness, drowsiness, dizziness, dyspnea).

Test renal and audiometric function frequently.

I-173

AMINOGLYCOSIDES ⟷ CURARIFORM DRUGS

278 510 704   512 800 802
396 538

Reaction: Additive neuromuscular blockade; respiratory depression progressing to apnea can result.

Suggestion: When giving curariform drugs during or following aminoglycoside therapy, observe patients closely for evidence of respiratory depression.

I-175

AMINOGLYCOSIDES ⟷ POLYMYXINS

278 510 704   196 198 450
396 538

Reactions: 1. Additive nephrotoxicity.
                 2. Possible additive neuromuscular depression.

Suggestions: If this combination is unavoidable, monitor renal function, and watch for evidence of nephrotoxicity (hematuria, oliguria, polydipsia, anorexia, nausea, vomiting, weakness, drowsiness, dizziness, dyspnea) and neuromuscular depression (respiratory difficulty, skeletal muscle weakness).

Note: Topical use of these agents can cause the same reactions.

AMINOGLYCOSIDES ⟷ VANCOMYCIN

278 510 704   560
396 538

Reaction: Additive ototoxicity and nephrotoxicity. Ototoxic effects can be severe and permanent.

Suggestions: Avoid this combination if possible. When combined therapy is unavoidable, monitor patients for evidence of ototoxicity (dizziness, vertigo, tinnitus, nausea, vomiting, hearing loss) and nephrotoxicity (hematuria, oliguria, polydipsia, anorexia, nausea, vomiting, weakness, drowsiness, dizziness, dyspnea).

Test renal and audiometric function frequently.

AMINOGLYCOSIDES ⟷ VIOMYCIN

278 510 704   564
396 538

Reaction: Additive ototoxicity and nephrotoxicity. Ototoxic effects can be severe and permanent.

Suggestions: Try to avoid this combination. When it cannot be avoided, monitor patients for evidence of ototoxicity (dizziness, vertigo, tinnitus, nausea, vomiting, hearing loss) and nephrotoxicity (hematuria, oliguria, polydipsia, anorexia, nausea, vomiting, weakness, drowsiness, dizziness, dyspnea).

Test renal and audiometric function frequently.

PARA-AMINO-SALICYLIC ACID ⟷ DIPHENHYDRAMINE

118   226

Reaction: Diphenhydramine interferes with gastric absorption of para-aminosalicylic acid, possibly diminishing its effect.

Suggestion: Give para-aminosalicylic acid at least 1 hour before or 2 hours after diphenhydramine.

I-183

PARA-AMINO-   ⟷   PROBENECID
SALICYLIC ACID
118   458

Reaction: Increase in serum levels of para-aminosalicylic acid, possibly leading to toxicity. Toxic effects may include severe nausea, vomiting, diarrhea.

Suggestion: If this combination is unavoidable, reduce para-aminosalicylic acid dosage by 50%.

Note: Para-aminosalicylic acid is rarely used today because of its toxicity.

I-185

PARA-AMINO-   ⟷   RIFAMPIN
SALICYLIC ACID
118   490

Reaction: Para-aminosalicylic acid products can significantly reduce the absorption of rifampin.

Suggestion: If these drugs must be given concurrently, separate the doses by 6 hours.

I-187

AMPHETAMINES   ⟷   PHENOTHIAZINES/
                             BUTYROPHENONES

138   706   174   370   472
                             260   466   758
                             290   468   848

Reaction: Possible decreased anorectic effect of amphetamine.

Suggestion: Avoid this combination, if anorectic amphetamine effect is desired.

Note: Phenothiazines have been used in the treatment of amphetamine overdosage.

AMPHETAMINES   ⟷   URINARY ALKALINIZERS

138   706

104   336   726
332   500   728
334   722   782

Reaction: Enhanced amphetamine effect from increased renal tubular absorption of amphetamine. Increased CNS stimulation and toxicity can result. Toxic effects may include nervousness and irritability, dryness of mouth, blurred vision, dizziness, palpitations, hypertension, cardiac arrhythmias, and hypertonic movements of head, neck, extremities.

Suggestions: Avoid concurrent use of amphetamines and urinary alkalinizers, such as antacids.

If this combination is unavoidable and must be continued for a prolonged period, monitor urinary pH, and advise patients to promptly report any toxic symptoms.

Alkalinizing diets (high in dairy products, vegetables, citrus juices, nuts) may also cause a reaction.

PHENYTOIN AND OTHER HYDANTOINS   ⟷   VALPROIC ACID

446   824

558

Reactions: 1. Increased risk of phenytoin toxicity due to possible rise in free serum phenytoin via its displacement from protein-bound sites. Toxic effects may include ataxia, nystagmus, diplopia.
2. Possible additive CNS depression.

Suggestions: 1. Anticipate possible need to reduce phenytoin dosage. Decision must usually be based on clinical judgment; only a few laboratories measure "free phenytoin" levels. (Conventional measurements of phenytoin levels are not helpful.)
2. See Interaction #I-435.

Note: These other hydantoins may react the same way: #824 ethotoin and #824 mephenytoin.

I-193

ANABOLIC STEROIDS ⟷ ANTIDIABETIC
AGENTS

708

176 544

304 826

Reaction: Possible increased hypoglycemic effect. Symptoms of
hypoglycemia include faintness, weakness, sweating, palpitations,
tachycardia, headache, confusion, ataxia, visual disturbances.

Suggestions: Closely monitor urine and blood sugar during
combined therapy and after stopping the anabolic steroid. Adjust
antidiabetic dosage accordingly.

Advise patients to promptly report any hypoglycemic symptoms.
Also advise patients to keep a candy bar, sugar cube, or other
source of simple carbohydrate readily available for emergencies.

I-195

SULFONAMIDES ⟷ THIOPENTAL

514 522 872

516 526

532

Reaction: Increase in thiopental levels, possibly leading to toxicity.
Respiratory depression can result.

Suggestion: Pay particular attention to maintaining respiratory
adequacy when using thiopental in patients taking sulfonamides.

I-197

ANABOLIC AND ⟷ ANTICOAGULANTS,
ANDROGENIC   ORAL
STEROIDS

708 712

140 742

568 744

Reaction: Increased anticoagulant effect.

Suggestions: When adding anabolic or androgenic steroids, reduce
anticoagulant dosage by $\frac{1}{3}$ and monitor prothrombin time
frequently. Readjust dosage of anticoagulant after steroid is
stopped.

Instruct patients to promptly report any unusual bruising or bleeding (such as bleeding gums, blood in urine, unusually heavy menstrual periods, rectal bleeding, black or tarry stools).

Topical vaginal application of androgenic steroids may also cause a reaction.

GENERAL ANESTHETICS, INHALATION	⟷	LINCOMYCIN/ CLINDAMYCIN
270 372		184
292 716		324

Reaction: Possible increased neuromuscular blockade and respiratory depression. (This most commonly occurs with cyclopropane or the halogenated hydrocarbons. It does *not* occur with ether or nitrous oxide.)

Suggestions: When administering inhalation anesthetics to patients who have been taking lincomycin or clindamycin, pay particular attention to maintaining respiratory adequacy. Use caution when giving either antibiotic during or following inhalation anesthesia.

CALCIUM BLOCKERS	⟷	DIGOXIN
910		224

Reaction: Verapamil can increase serum digoxin levels by as much as 50%. Nifedipine (another calcium blocker) may affect digoxin similarly, but to a lesser degree.

Digoxin toxicity can result. Symptoms may include anorexia, nausea and vomiting, confusion, blurred vision, photophobia, unusual fatigue or weakness, headache, bradycardia or tachycardia, arrhythmias.

Suggestions: When adding verapamil, a $\frac{1}{3}$ reduction in digoxin dosage may be needed. Measure digoxin blood level, and adjust dosage accordingly.

When adding nifedipine, monitor patients for clinical toxicity, measure digoxin blood level, and adjust dosage if required.

Advise patients to promptly report any toxic symptoms.

I-203

PHENOBARBITAL   ⟷   VALPROIC ACID

434   558

Reaction: Increased phenobarbital plasma levels and effect, via inhibited phenobarbital metabolism. Excessive sedation can result.

Suggestions: When these drugs must be given together, reduce phenobarbital dosage by ½, and monitor plasma levels of phenobarbital, further adjusting dosage as indicated. Anticipate the need to increase phenobarbital dosage when valproic acid is stopped.

I-205

SALICYLATES   ⟷   URINARY ALKALINIZERS

112	866	104	336	726
		332	500	728
		334	722	782

Reaction: Urinary alkalinization increases renal elimination of salicylates, resulting in reduced salicylate levels and effects.

Suggestions: In patients taking large doses of salicylates (eg, for arthritis or rheumatic fever), monitor plasma salicylate levels, and watch for reduced effectiveness of therapy. Anticipate increased salicylate dosage requirements when adding alkalinizing agents and decreased requirements when stopping them.

Alkalinizing diets (high in dairy products, vegetables, citrus juices, nuts) may also cause a reaction.

I-207

GENERAL ANESTHETICS, INHALATION   ⟷   POLYMYXINS

270	372	196	198	450
292	716			

Reaction: Additive neuromuscular depression, principally affecting respiration, after intraperitoneal use of polymyxin (especially if a curariform drug is also given).

Suggestion: Observe patients closely for evidence of respiratory depression.

SALICYLATES   ⟷   SULFINPYRAZONE

112   866   524

Reactions: 1. Additive gastric irritation with possible bleeding.
                  2. Inhibition of sulfinpyrazone uricosuric effect.
                  3. With large salicylate doses (equivalent to, or greater than, 3.5 gm of aspirin per day), salicylism is possible via reduced renal salicylate excretion. Symptoms may include tinnitus, dizziness, hearing loss, vomiting, restlessness, delirium, lethargy, hyperpnea, and burning in mouth, throat, abdomen.

Suggestion: Avoid large doses of salicylates during sulfinpyrazone therapy. Occasional analgesic doses are unlikely to cause reactions.

Note: Pepto-Bismol (bismuth subsalicylate) is an unexpected source of significant amounts of salicylate.

ANTACIDS   ⟷   BETA BLOCKERS

332	500	726		382	476
334	722	728		392	776
336					

Reaction: Antacids can interfere with oral absorption of beta blockers, decreasing their effect. Exception: The absorption of #382 metoprolol is not affected.

Suggestion: Give beta blocker at least 1 hour before or 2 hours after antacid.

ANTACIDS   ⟷   DIGOXIN

332   722   224
334   726
336   728

Reactions: Antacids (other than sodium bicarbonate) can interfere with oral absorption of digoxin, possibly decreasing its effect.

continued

I-213
continued

Antacids with laxative effects (magnesium salts: #332, #334, #336) can also cause hypokalemia, which increases the sensitivity of the myocardium to digoxin and may increase digitalis cardiotoxicity.

Suggestions: Give digoxin at least 1 hour before or 2 hours after any antacid.

Advise patients to report any prolonged diarrhea. See Interaction #I-537 regarding hypokalemia.

I-215

ANTACIDS	⟷	IRON SALTS

332	500	726	830
334	722	728	
336			

Reaction: Antacids (especially #728 magnesium trisilicate) can interfere with oral iron absorption, decreasing its effect.

Suggestion: If this combination is unavoidable, space iron and antacid doses as far apart as possible.

I-217

ANTACIDS/LAXATIVES ⟷ TETRACYCLINES
WITH METALLIC
CATIONS

332	336	722	728		240	416
334	500	726	834		386	880

Reaction: Antacids and those laxatives that contain metallic cations (aluminum, magnesium, calcium) can decrease oral tetracycline absorption by 50-100%. Decreased tetracycline effect is likely.

Suggestions: Avoid simultaneous doses of these agents. Give tetracycline at least 2 hours before or 3 hours after any antacid or laxative with number listed above.

See Food Interaction #F-16.

ANTACIDS—   ⟷   ISONIAZID
ALUMINUM

722   310

Reaction: Decreased absorption of oral isoniazid; possible decreased effect.

Suggestion: Give isoniazid 1–2 hours before any aluminum antacid.

ANTACIDS—   ⟷ PHENOTHIAZINES
ALUMINUM, CALCIUM,
MAGNESIUM

332	722	174	466	758
334	726	260	468	848
336	728	370	472	

Reaction: Possible decreased absorption of oral phenothiazine.

Suggestion: Separate doses of these agents by 2 or more hours.

ANTACIDS—CALCIUM,   ⟷ SODIUM
MAGNESIUM   POLYSTYRENE
                            SULFONATE RESIN

332	336	728	506
334	726		

Reactions: Metabolic alkalosis. Symptoms may include irritability and neuromuscular stimulation, possibly progressing to tetany.

If secondary hypokalemia occurs, the following symptoms may result: muscular weakness with hypoventilation, diminished GI motility with bloating that can progress to paralytic ileus, polyuria, general weakness, hypotension with dizziness, light-headedness, and faintness.

Suggestions: Advise patients to promptly report any of the above symptoms, so that dosage adjustment can be made or medications changed.

Rectal administration of sodium polystyrene sulfonate resin may minimize the problem.

I-225
ANTACIDS— ⟷ DICUMAROL
ALUMINUM,
MAGNESIUM

332   336   728   **140**
334   722

Reaction: Possible increased absorption and effect of dicumarol.

Suggestion: Monitor prothrombin time more closely than usual, and adjust dicumarol dosage accordingly.

I-227
HYPOGLYCEMICS, ⟷ RIFAMPIN
ORAL

176   544   826   **490**

Reaction: Decreased hypoglycemic effect.

Suggestion: Monitor urine and blood sugar both during and following combined therapy. Adjust hypoglycemic dosage accordingly.

I-229
ANTIANGINAL ⟷ VASODILATORS
AGENTS   (OTHER)

316   402   730   **418   542   896**
382   476   776
392

Reaction: Additive hypotension. Postural hypotension (dizziness, light-headedness, weakness) may progress to syncope. Severe hypotension can progress to seizures and shock.

Suggestions: Use this combination with caution.

Advise patients to lie down immediately, rest, then change position slowly if early symptoms of postural hypotension occur. Also advise patients to promptly report any of the above symptoms, so that dosage adjustment can be made or medications changed.

ANTIANGINALS/ $\longleftrightarrow$ ANTIHYPERTENSIVES
ANTIARRHYTHMICS

132	402	190	350	438	616
230	460	218	376	452	760
246	730	254	382	476	776
316	732	276	388	504	820
322	862	296	392	508	864
		342	436	546	882

Reactions: **1.** Additive hypotension. Postural hypotension (dizziness, light-headedness, weakness) may progress to syncope. Severe hypotension can progress to seizures and shock.
2. If procainamide (#460) is combined with reserpine or a related drug (#864), cardiotoxicity with arrhythmias can result.
3. If IV lidocaine (#322) is given with propranolol (#476), decreased lidocaine metabolism and up to $\frac{1}{3}$ increase in plasma levels of lidocaine may result, possibly leading to toxicity. Toxic effects may include CNS depression, depression of myocardial contractility.

Suggestions: **1.** Use this combination with caution. Advise patients to lie down immediately, rest, then change position slowly if early symptoms of postural hypotension occur.
2. Do not start procainamide until at least 24 hours after starting a reserpine-type drug. Start with small doses, and monitor closely for arrhythmias.
3. When giving IV lidocaine with propranolol, carefully monitor patients for evidence of lidocaine toxicity. Lidocaine dosage reduction may be appropriate.

DIGOXIN $\longleftrightarrow$ QUINIDINE/QUININE

224   862

Reaction: Approximate doubling of serum digoxin levels within first 2–5 days after beginning quinidine. GI side effects and risk of cardiac arrhythmias are frequently increased.

continued

I-233

continued

Suggestions: When starting quinidine in patients on maintenance digoxin therapy, reduce digoxin dosage by 50%. Measure serum digoxin levels after 4–5 days, and adjust digoxin dosage accordingly.

Advise patients to promptly report any early signs of digitalis toxicity: anorexia, nausea and vomiting, confusion, blurred vision, photophobia, unusual fatigue or weakness, headache, bradycardia or tachycardia, arrhythmias.

Note: Quinine, the levo-stereo isomer of quinidine, appears to affect digoxin in a similar manner but to a lesser degree.

I-235

ANTICHOLINERGICS, ⟷ ANTICHOLINERGIC-
CENTRALLY ACTING   LIKE CNS
                       DEPRESSANTS

| 172 | 260 | 408 | 550 |
| 226 | 284 | 492 | 736 |

174	466	768
290	468	848
298	472	884
330	756	888
370	758	

Reactions: 1. Additive anticholinergic side effects: ataxia, blurred vision, constipation, dizziness, dry mouth, gastric irritation, palpitations, slurred speech, toxic psychosis (agitation, delirium, disorientation), urinary retention.
2. Additive CNS depression.

Suggestions: 1. While there are indications for this combination, additive side effects must be anticipated. Use the lowest possible dose of each drug, and advise patients to promptly report any side effects.

Avoid using any anticholinergic drug in patients with glaucoma.
2. See Interaction #I-435.

ANTICHOLINERGICS, ⟷ LEVODOPA
ALL

132	226	374	550	320
136	260	408	736	
172	284	470	738	
220	312	492		

Reactions: 1. Decreased levodopa effect.
2. Additive anticholinergic side effects: ataxia, blurred vision, constipation, dizziness, dry mouth, gastric irritation, palpitations, slurred speech, toxic psychosis (agitation, delirium, disorientation), urinary retention.

Suggestions: 1. Monitor clinical effect of levodopa, and adjust its dosage accordingly, both during combined therapy and after stopping the anticholinergic.
2. Advise patients to promptly report any side effects.

Avoid using any anticholinergic drug in patients with glaucoma.

Note: Levodopa-carbidopa (Sinemet) produces a higher concentration of levodopa with milder, less frequent side effects.

ANTICHOLINERGICS, ⟷ ANTICHOLINERGIC-
CENTRALLY ACTING LIKE DRUGS WITHOUT
CNS DEPRESSANT
ACTIVITY

172	260	408	550	114	230	862
226	284	492	736			

Reaction: Additive anticholinergic side effects: ataxia, blurred vision, constipation, dizziness, dry mouth, gastric irritation, palpitations, slurred speech, toxic psychosis (agitation, delirium, disorientation), urinary retention.

Suggestions: Anticipate additive effects, and use lowest possible dose of each drug.

Advise patients to promptly report any side effects. Dosage reduction or change of medication may be necessary.

Avoid using any anticholinergic drug in patients with glaucoma.

I-241

ANTICHOLINERGICS, ⟷ ANTICHOLINERGICS,
CENTRALLY ACTING   CENTRALLY ACTING

(Every drug with number listed below interacts with every other drug in the list.)

172	260	408	550
226	284	492	736

Reactions: 1. Additive anticholinergic side effects: ataxia, blurred vision, constipation, dizziness, dry mouth, gastric irritation, palpitations, slurred speech, toxic psychosis (agitation, delirium, disorientation), urinary retention.
2. Additive CNS depression.

Suggestions: 1. While there are indications for this combination, additive side effects must be anticipated. Use the lowest possible dose of each drug, and advise patients to promptly report any side effects.

Avoid using any anticholinergic drug in patients with glaucoma.

2. See Interaction #I-435.

I-243

ANTICHOLINERGICS, ⟷ ANTICHOLINERGICS,
CENTRALLY ACTING   PERIPHERALLY
ACTING

172	260	408	550		132	220	374	738
226	284	492	736		136	312	470	

Reaction: Additive anticholinergic side effects: ataxia, blurred vision, constipation, dizziness, dry mouth, gastric irritation, palpitations, slurred speech, toxic psychosis (agitation, delirium, disorientation), urinary retention.

Suggestions: Anticipate additive effects, and use lowest possible dose of each drug.

Advise patients to promptly report any side effects. Dosage reduction or change of medication may be necessary.

Avoid using any anticholinergic drug in patients with glaucoma.

RESERPINE AND   ⟷   TRICYCLIC
RELATED DRUGS   ANTIDEPRESSANTS

864   888

Reaction: Possible CNS stimulation with hyperexcitability and mania.

Suggestions: Avoid using reserpine for antihypertensive therapy in patients taking tricyclic antidepressants.

Reserve the reserpine-tricyclic combination for therapy of severe depression in refractory patients, and closely monitor for excessive CNS stimulation.

Note: The following drugs are chemically related to reserpine and will cause the same reaction: #864 alseroxylon; #864 deserpidine; #864 rauwolfia serpentina (whole root rauwolfia); #864 rescinnamine; #864 syrosingopine.

QUINIDINE/QUININE ⟷ URINARY
                                    ALKALINIZERS

862   104   336   726

                              332   500   728

                              334   722   782

Reaction: Alkalinization of the urine increases renal reabsorption of quinidine and may cause toxicity. Toxic effects may include ventricular arrhythmias, cinchonism (headache, palpitations, dizziness, visual disturbances, tinnitus).

Suggestions: Patients on alkalinizing drugs or diets (high in dairy products, vegetables, citrus juices, nuts) may require reduction of quinidine dosage. (See Food Interaction #F-14.)

Advise patients to report any symptoms of cinchonism or changes in pulse.

Note: Quinine (#862) is chemically related to quinidine and may react the same way.

I-249

CORTICOSTEROIDS $\longleftrightarrow$ PHENYTOIN AND
OTHER HYDANTOINS

202	**266**	**446**
210	**798**	**824**

Reactions: **1.** Increased corticosteroid metabolism, possibly resulting in decreased therapeutic response.
   2. Dexamethasone (#798) in high doses may inhibit the metabolism of phenytoin.

Suggestions: **1.** Carefully monitor therapeutic response to corticosteroid when adding phenytoin. If phenytoin must be continued, corticosteroid dosage may have to be increased.
   2. Monitor serum phenytoin levels during concurrent therapy with dexamethasone.

Note: These other hydantoins may cause the same reaction: #824 ethotoin and #824 mephenytoin.

I-251

MONOAMINE OXIDASE $\longleftrightarrow$ TRICYCLIC
INHIBITORS AND   ANTIDEPRESSANTS
RELATED DRUGS

274   464   836   **888**

Reaction: Possible severe hyperexcitability, hyperpyrexia, convulsions. Deaths have occurred.

Suggestions: Avoid except under carefully controlled conditions in refractory patients unresponsive to safer therapy. The safest combination therapy, if it must be used, is isocarboxazid or phenelzine t.i.d. in daytime, with amitriptyline at bedtime. Warn patients to seek immediate medical help if severe headache suddenly develops.

When switching from a tricyclic antidepressant to an MAO inhibitor, allow at least a 14-day hiatus between drugs.

Note: The following drugs are chemically related to MAO inhibitors and can cause the same reaction: #274 furazolidone and #464 procarbazine.

ANTICHOLINERGICS, ⟷ ANTICHOLINERGICS,
PERIPHERALLY   PERIPHERALLY
ACTING   ACTING

(Every drug with number listed below interacts with every other drug in the list.)

132	220	374	738
136	312	470	

Reaction: Additive anticholinergic side effects: ataxia, blurred vision, constipation, dizziness, dry mouth, gastric irritation, palpitations, slurred speech, toxic psychosis (agitation, delirium, disorientation), urinary retention.

Suggestions: Anticipate additive effects, and use lowest possible dose of each drug.

Advise patients to promptly report any side effects. Dosage reduction or change of medication may be necessary.

Avoid using any anticholinergic drug in patients with glaucoma.

ANTICHOLINERGICS, ⟷ ANTICHOLINERGIC-
PERIPHERALLY   LIKE DRUGS
ACTING

132	312	470		114	330	472	848
136	374	738		174	370	756	862
220				230	466	758	884
				290	468	768	888
				298			

Reaction: Additive anticholinergic side effects: ataxia, blurred vision, constipation, dizziness, dry mouth, gastric irritation, palpitations, slurred speech, toxic psychosis (agitation, delirium, disorientation), urinary retention.

Suggestions: Anticipate additive effects, and use lowest possible dose of each drug.

Advise patients to promptly report any side effects. Dosage reduction or change of medication may be necessary.

Avoid using any anticholinergic drug in patients with glaucoma.

I-257

ANTICOAGULANTS,   ⟷   TETRACYCLINES
ORAL

| 140 | 742 | 240 | 416 |
| 568 | 744 | 386 | 880 |

Reaction: Possible increased anticoagulant effect (seen with #240 doxycycline, but high doses of other tetracyclines may also cause this reaction).

Suggestion: Monitor prothrombin time frequently, and adjust anticoagulant dosage accordingly, both during and following concurrent therapy.

I-259

ANTICOAGULANTS,   ⟷   SULFINPYRAZONE
ORAL

| 140 | 742 | 524 |
| 568 | 744 | |

Reaction: Increased anticoagulant effect and risk of hemorrhage.

Suggestions: Marked prolongation of prothrombin time and development of major hemorrhage have been reported in anticoagulated patients given sulfinpyrazone. Therefore, it seems advisable to reduce anticoagulant dosage by 25% when starting sulfinpyrazone.

Monitor prothrombin time frequently, and adjust anticoagulant dosage accordingly, both during and following concurrent therapy.

I-261

COUMARIN   ⟷   CIMETIDINE
ANTICOAGULANTS

| 140 | 568 | 742 | 180 |

Reaction: Possible increased anticoagulant effect.

Suggestions: Monitor prothrombin time frequently, and adjust anticoagulant dosage accordingly, both during and following concurrent therapy.

Instruct patients to promptly report any unusual bruising or bleeding (such as bleeding gums, blood in urine, unusually heavy menstrual periods, rectal bleeding, black or tarry stools).

DICUMAROL   ⟷   PHENYTOIN AND
OTHER HYDANTOINS

140   446   824

Reactions: **1.** Increase in serum phenytoin levels, possibly
leading to toxicity. Toxic effects may include
ataxia, nystagmus, diplopia.
             2. Decrease in serum dicumarol levels with
corresponding decrease in prothrombin time.

Suggestions: **1.** Advise patients to promptly report any symptoms
of phenytoin toxicity. Measure serum phenytoin
levels approximately 1 week after starting
dicumarol, and adjust phenytoin dosage if needed.
             2. Closely monitor prothrombin time both during
and following concurrent therapy, and adjust
anticoagulant dosage accordingly.

Note: While this interaction is usually described as Dicumarol-
Phenytoin, the other hydantoins (#824 ethotoin and #824
mephenytoin) can probably cause the same reactions.

ALLOPURINOL   ⟷   THEOPHYLLINE AND
OTHER XANTHINES

110   902

Reaction: Long-term allopurinol therapy may decrease theophylline
metabolism and increase its serum levels, possibly leading to
toxicity. Toxic effects may include GI upset with nausea and
vomiting, headache, irritability, dizziness, tremors, insomnia,
seizures, tachycardia, cardiac arrhythmias.

Suggestions: Measure serum theophylline levels after 2 weeks of
combined therapy, and adjust theophylline dosage accordingly.

Advise patients to promptly report any toxic symptoms.

Note: These other xanthines may react the same way: #902
aminophylline; #902 oxtriphylline. Dyphylline (#902) is excreted
as unchanged drug in the urine and is unlikely to interact.

I-267

ANTICOAGULANTS, ORAL	⟷	BARBITURATES/ PRIMIDONE

140	742		366	456	532
568	744		430	494	588
			434	530	772

Reaction: Decreased anticoagulant effect via barbiturate dose-dependent induction of hepatic microsomal enzymes that increase anticoagulant metabolism.

Suggestions: Monitor prothrombin time weekly. Anticipate the need for a 25–60% increase in anticoagulant dosage when barbiturate is started, and a dosage reduction about 2 weeks after barbiturate is stopped to avoid over-anticoagulation and hemorrhage.

Advise patients to promptly report any unusual bruising or bleeding (such as bleeding gums, blood in urine, unusually heavy menstrual periods, rectal bleeding, black or tarry stools), especially after barbiturate has been stopped.

Note: Primidone (#456) is metabolized to phenobarbital and will cause the same reaction.

I-269

ANTICOAGULANTS, ORAL	⟷	CARBAMAZEPINE

140	742		150
568	744		

Reaction: Markedly decreased anticoagulant effect, as carbamazepine increases hepatic metabolism of anticoagulants.

Suggestions: Monitor prothrombin time weekly, and increase anticoagulant dosage as needed.

When stopping carbamazepine, continue to monitor prothrombin time. Anticipate the need to decrease anticoagulant dosage after about 2 weeks to avoid over-anticoagulation and hemorrhage.

Advise patients to promptly report any unusual bruising or bleeding (such as bleeding gums, blood in urine, unusually heavy menstrual periods, rectal bleeding, black or tarry stools), especially after carbamazepine has been stopped.

ANTICOAGULANTS, ⟷ CHLORAL
ORAL DERIVATIVES/
TRICLOFOS

| 140 | 742 | 548 | 790 |
| 568 | 744 | | |

Reaction: Possible temporary increase in anticoagulant effect.

Suggestions: Advise patients to promptly report any unusual bruising or bleeding (such as bleeding gums, blood in urine, unusually heavy menstrual periods, rectal bleeding, black or tarry stools).

There is evidence that this interaction is of little clinical importance, and that the usual precautions in monitoring anticoagulant therapy are sufficient.

Alternative drugs that do not interact are available (eg, benzodiazepines, such as chlordiazepoxide, clorazepate, diazepam).

Note: Triclofos (#548) is chemically related to chloral derivatives and can cause the same reaction.

ANTICOAGULANTS, ⟷ CHLORAMPHENICOL
ORAL

| 140 | 742 | 166 |
| 568 | 744 | |

Reaction: Possible increased anticoagulant effect, mainly with dicumarol.

Suggestions: Monitor prothrombin time frequently, and adjust anticoagulant dosage accordingly, both during and following concurrent therapy.

Advise patients to promptly report any unusual bruising or bleeding (such as bleeding gums, blood in urine, unusually heavy menstrual periods, rectal bleeding, black or tarry stools).

I-275

ANTICOAGULANTS, ⟷ CHOLESTYRAMINE
ORAL

140 **742** **178**
568 **744**

Reaction: Decreased anticoagulant absorption and effect.

Suggestions: When combination therapy is unavoidable, give cholestyramine at least 3 hours (preferably 6 hours) after the anticoagulant.

Monitor prothrombin time frequently, and adjust anticoagulant dosage accordingly, both during and following concurrent therapy.

Advise patients to promptly report any unusual bruising or bleeding (such as bleeding gums, blood in urine, unusually heavy menstrual periods, rectal bleeding, black or tarry stools), especially after cholestyramine has been stopped.

I-277

ANTICOAGULANTS, ⟷ CLOFIBRATE
ORAL

140 **742** **186**
568 **744**

Reaction: Increased anticoagulant effect, most likely in patients who are hyperlipidemic, and who sustain a reduction in serum lipids from clofibrate therapy.

Suggestions: Because a substantial increase in anticoagulation is possible, an anticoagulant dosage reduction of $\frac{1}{3}$ is advisable when starting clofibrate.

Monitor prothrombin time frequently, and adjust anticoagulant dosage accordingly, both during and following concurrent therapy.

Advise patients to promptly report any unusual bruising or bleeding (such as bleeding gums, blood in urine, unusually heavy menstrual periods, rectal bleeding, black or tarry stools).

ANTICOAGULANTS,   ↔   CONTRACEPTIVES,
ORAL   ORAL/ESTROGENS

140	742		404	584	816
568	744		576	586	860

Reaction: Possible increased anticoagulant effect.

Suggestions: Monitor prothrombin time frequently, and adjust anticoagulant dosage accordingly, both during and following concurrent therapy.

Advise patients to promptly report any unusual bruising or bleeding (such as bleeding gums, blood in urine, unusually heavy menstrual periods, rectal bleeding, black or tarry stools).

Note: This interaction may not occur with contraceptives that contain only progestogens: #404 norethindrone (Micronor, Nor-Q.D.), or #576 norgestrel (Ovrette).

ANTICOAGULANTS,   ↔   CORTICOSTEROIDS
ORAL

140	742		202	266
568	744		210	798

Reactions: **1.** Possible decreased anticoagulant effect.
                 2. Possible increased risk of hemorrhage by "stress-like" impairment of vascular/platelet function.
                 3. Possible increased risk of corticosteroid-induced GI ulceration with risk of bleeding.

Suggestions: Monitor prothrombin time frequently, and adjust anticoagulant dosage accordingly, both during and following concurrent therapy.

Advise patients to promptly report any unusual bruising or bleeding (such as bleeding gums, blood in urine, unusually heavy menstrual periods, rectal bleeding, black or tarry stools).

Warn patients of ulcer-forming potential of corticosteroids. Advise them to promptly report any upper abdominal pain, especially if related to eating; or unusual tiredness or weakness.

Note: Applying large quantities of high-potency *topical* corticosteroids may result in significant absorption and systemic activity.

I-283

ANTICOAGULANTS,   ⟷   DISULFIRAM
ORAL

140 742   232
568 744

Reaction: Increased anticoagulant effect.

Suggestions: Monitor prothrombin time frequently, and adjust anticoagulant dosage accordingly, both during and following concurrent therapy. Anticipate the need for decreased anticoagulant dosage when starting disulfiram and increased dosage when stopping it.

Advise patients to promptly report any unusual bruising or bleeding (such às bleeding gums, blood in urine, unusually heavy menstrual periods, rectal bleeding, black or tarry stools).

I-285

ANTICOAGULANTS,   ⟷   ETHACRYNIC ACID
ORAL

140 742   254
568 744

Reactions: 1. Possible increased anticoagulant effect.
               2. Possible GI ulceration.

Suggestions: 1. If combined therapy is unavoidable, monitor prothrombin time frequently (daily, if ethacrynic acid is given IV), and adjust anticoagulant dosage accordingly, both during and following concurrent therapy. Anticipate the need for decreased anticoagulant dosage when starting ethacrynic acid and increased dosage when stopping it.

              Advise patients to promptly report any unusual bruising or bleeding (such as bleeding gums, blood in urine, unusually heavy menstrual periods, rectal bleeding, black or tarry stools).
      2. Advise patients to promptly report any unusual tiredness or weakness, or upper abdominal pain (especially if related to eating).

ANTICOAGULANTS, ⟷ ETHCHLORVYNOL
ORAL

| 140 | 742 | 256 |
| 568 | 744 | |

Reaction: Possible decreased anticoagulant effect.

Suggestions: Monitor prothrombin time frequently, and adjust anticoagulant dosage accordingly, both during and following concurrent therapy. Anticipate the need for significantly increased anticoagulant dosage 1–2 weeks after starting ethchlorvynol, and decreased dosage 1–2 weeks after stopping it.

Note: Alternative sedatives that do not interact include benzodiazepines, such as chlordiazepoxide, clorazepate, diazepam.

ANTICOAGULANTS, ⟷ GLUCAGON
ORAL

| 140 | 742 | 280 |
| 568 | 744 | |

Reaction: Increased anticoagulant effect (glucagon dose-related).

Suggestions: Monitor prothrombin time frequently, and adjust anticoagulant dosage accordingly, both during and following concurrent therapy.

Advise patients to promptly report any unusual bruising or bleeding (such as bleeding gums, blood in urine, unusually heavy menstrual periods, rectal bleeding, black or tarry stools).

ANTICOAGULANTS, ⟷ GLUTETHIMIDE
ORAL

| 140 | 742 | 282 |
| 568 | 744 | |

Reaction: Decreased anticoagulant effect.

Suggestions: Monitor prothrombin time frequently, and adjust anticoagulant dosage accordingly, both during and following concurrent therapy. Anticipate the need for increased anticoagulant dosage when starting glutethimide and decreased dosage when stopping it.

continued

I-291
continued

Advise patients to promptly report any unusual bruising or
bleeding (such as bleeding gums, blood in urine, unusually heavy
menstrual periods, rectal bleeding, black or tarry stools), especially
after glutethimide has been stopped.

I-293
ANTICOAGULANTS,   ⟷   GRISEOFULVIN
ORAL

140	742	288
568	744	

Reaction: Decreased anticoagulant effect.

Suggestions: Monitor prothrombin time frequently, and adjust
anticoagulant dosage accordingly, both during and following
concurrent therapy. Anticipate the need for significantly increased
anticoagulant dosage when starting griseofulvin and decreased
dosage when stopping it.

Advise patients to promptly report any unusual bruising or
bleeding (such as bleeding gums, blood in urine, unusually heavy
menstrual periods, rectal bleeding, black or tarry stools), especially
after griseofulvin has been stopped.

I-295
ANTICOAGULANTS,   ⟷   INDOMETHACIN
ORAL

140	742	302
568	744	

Reactions: 1. Possible increased anticoagulant effect and risk of
hemorrhage.
2. Increased risk of indomethacin-induced GI
ulceration.

Suggestions: Try to avoid using indomethacin in anticoagulated
patients. Alternative nonsteroidal anti-inflammatory agents are
available that cause less gastric irritation and do not increase
anticoagulant effects (eg, ibuprofen, naproxen).

If combined therapy is unavoidable, monitor prothrombin time
frequently, and adjust anticoagulant dosage accordingly, both
during and following concurrent therapy. Anticipate the need for
decreased anticoagulant dosage when starting indomethacin and
increased dosage when stopping it.

Advise patients to promptly report any unusual bruising or bleeding, abdominal pain, black or tarry stools, unusual tiredness or weakness.

ANTICOAGULANTS,   ⟷   MEFENAMIC ACID
ORAL

140	**742**	**344**	
568	**744**		

Reactions: 1. Increased anticoagulant effect and risk of hemorrhage.
2. Increased risk of mefenamic acid-induced gastric irritation and ulceration.

Suggestion: Avoid this combination. Alternatives can usually be found for mefenamic acid.

ANTICOAGULANTS,   ⟷   METRONIDAZOLE
ORAL

140	**742**	**384**	
568	**744**		

Reaction: Increased anticoagulant effect and risk of hemorrhage.

Suggestions: Because this combination has caused significant prolongation of prothrombin time and major hemorrhage, it seems advisable to reduce anticoagulant dosage by 50% when starting metronidazole, and to measure prothrombin time every 3 days, making further dosage adjustments as indicated.

An alternative possibility is to give a single 1.0 or 2.0 gm dose of metronidazole (for trichomonal infection) and to withhold the anticoagulant on the day of treatment.

Advise patients to promptly report any unusual bruising or bleeding (such as bleeding gums, blood in urine, unusually heavy menstrual periods, rectal bleeding, black or tarry stools).

I-301

ANTICOAGULANTS,   ⟷   NALIDIXIC ACID
ORAL

140   742   **394**
568   744

Reaction: Possible increased anticoagulant effect.

Suggestions: Monitor prothrombin time frequently, and adjust anticoagulant dosage accordingly, both during and following concurrent therapy.

Advise patients to promptly report any unusual bruising or bleeding (such as bleeding gums, blood in urine, unusually heavy menstrual periods, rectal bleeding, black or tarry stools).

I-303

ANTICOAGULANTS,   ⟷   OXYPHENBUTAZONE
ORAL

140   742   **414**
568   744

Reactions: 1. Markedly increased anticoagulant effect and risk of hemorrhage.
2. Increased risk of oxyphenbutazone-induced gastric irritation and ulceration.

Suggestion: Avoid this combination. Alternative nonsteroidal anti-inflammatory agents are available that cause less gastric irritation and do not increase anticoagulant effects (eg, ibuprofen, naproxen).

I-305

ANTICOAGULANTS,   ⟷   PHENYLBUTAZONE
ORAL

140   742   **440**
568   744

Reactions: 1. Markedly increased anticoagulant effect and risk of hemorrhage.
2. Increased risk of phenylbutazone-induced gastric irritation and ulceration.

Suggestion: Avoid this combination. Alternative nonsteroidal anti-inflammatory agents are available that cause less gastric irritation and do not increase anticoagulant effects (eg, ibuprofen, naproxen).

I-307

ANTICOAGULANTS, ⟷ ANTIHYPERTHYROID
ALL   AGENTS

140 568 744   **478 600**
294 742

Reaction: Possible increased anticoagulant effect associated with correction of hyperthyroidism.

Suggestions: Monitor prothrombin time (or Lee-White clotting time or activated partial thromboplastin time when using heparin), and adjust anticoagulant dosage accordingly, both during and following concurrent therapy.

Advise patients to promptly report any unusual bruising or bleeding (such as bleeding gums, blood in urine, unusually heavy menstrual periods, rectal bleeding, black or tarry stools).

I-309

ANTICOAGULANTS, ⟷ SULINDAC
ORAL

140 742   **606**
568 744

Reaction: Possible increased anticoagulant effect.

Suggestions: Monitor prothrombin time frequently, and adjust anticoagulant dosage accordingly, both during and following concurrent therapy. Anticipate the need for decreased anticoagulant dosage when starting sulindac and increased dosage when stopping it.

Advise patients to promptly report any unusual bruising or bleeding (such as bleeding gums, blood in urine, unusually heavy menstrual periods, rectal bleeding, black or tarry stools).

I-311

ANTICOAGULANTS,   ⟷   RIFAMPIN
ORAL

140	742	490
568	744	

Reaction: Markedly decreased anticoagulant effect.

Suggestions: Monitor prothrombin time frequently, and adjust anticoagulant dosage accordingly, both during and following concurrent therapy. Anticipate a possible need for a 50–100% increase in anticoagulant dosage when starting rifampin and a similar decrease when stopping it.

Advise patients to promptly report any unusual bruising or bleeding (such as bleeding gums, blood in urine, unusually heavy menstrual periods, rectal bleeding, black or tarry stools), especially after rifampin has been stopped.

I-313

ANTICOAGULANTS,   ⟷   SALICYLATES
ORAL

140	742	112 866
568	744	

Reactions:
1. Possible increased anticoagulant effect. (With aspirin, this occurs with doses in excess of 3 gm—10 5-grain tablets—per day.)
2. GI irritation with possible bleeding.
3. Aspirin alone inhibits platelet function, which may increase the risk of bleeding, even when used in small doses.

Suggestions: If salicylates are required, use magnesium salicylate, sodium salicylate, choline salicylate, salsalate, or salicylamide, as they are less likely than aspirin to cause reactions.

Acetaminophen is the usually recommended alternative to salicylates for analgesia.

If any salicylate is used, monitor prothrombin time frequently, and adjust anticoagulant dosage accordingly, both during and following concurrent therapy.

Advise patients to promptly report any unusual bruising or
bleeding (such as bleeding gums, blood in urine, unusually heavy
menstrual periods, rectal bleeding, black or tarry stools),
abdominal pain (especially if related to eating), unusual tiredness
or weakness.

Warn patients that many nonprescription drug products contain
aspirin. Advise them to seek professional advice before using any
cold or pain remedies.

Note: Pepto-Bismol (bismuth subsalicylate) is an unexpected source
of significant amounts of salicylate.

ANTICOAGULANTS,   ⟷   SULFONAMIDES
ORAL

| 140 | 742 | | 514 | 522 | 872 |
| 568 | 744 | | 516 | 526 | |

Reaction: Markedly increased anticoagulant effect.

Suggestions: When starting sulfonamides, reduce anticoagulant
dosage by 30%; when stopping sulfonamides, resume previous
anticoagulant maintenance dosage.

Monitor prothrombin time frequently, and adjust anticoagulant
dosage accordingly, both during and following concurrent therapy.

Advise patients to promptly report any unusual bruising or
bleeding (such as bleeding gums, blood in urine, unusually heavy
menstrual periods, rectal bleeding, black or tarry stools).

ANTICOAGULANTS,   ⟷   THYROID HORMONES/
ORAL   DEXTROTHYROXINE

| 140 | 742 | | 214 | 886 |
| 568 | 744 | | | |

Reactions:
1. Increased anticoagulant effect associated with correction of hypothyroidism. Dextrothyroxine (#214), used principally for lowering blood lipids, can have the same effect.
2. No effect in euthyroid patients on maintenance thyroid replacement.

continued

I-317
continued

Suggestions: Monitor prothrombin time frequently, and adjust anticoagulant dosage accordingly, both during and following concurrent therapy. Anticipate the need for decreased anticoagulant dosage when starting thyroid hormone and increased dosage when stopping it.

Advise patients to promptly report any unusual bruising or bleeding (such as bleeding gums, blood in urine, unusually heavy menstrual periods, rectal bleeding, black or tarry stools).

I-319

PROBENECID	←→	SALICYLATES
458		112 866

Reaction: Decreased uricosuric effect of probenecid.

Suggestion: Occasional doses of salicylates for analgesia are unlikely to inhibit uricosuria. The regular use of larger doses (more than 2.0 gm per day) should be avoided.

Note: Pepto-Bismol (bismuth subsalicylate) is an unexpected source of significant amounts of salicylate.

I-321

ANTICOAGULANTS, ORAL	←→	VITAMIN K
140 742		898
568 744		

Reaction: Decreased anticoagulant effect.

Suggestions: Restrict the use of vitamin K to the treatment of excessive anticoagulant activity.

Following large doses of vitamin K, patients may exhibit resistance to oral anticoagulants for several weeks. If larger anticoagulant doses are given to overcome this resistance, anticipate decreasing requirements as the vitamin K effect dissipates.

Notes: Day-to-day variations in vitamin K intake do not decrease anticoagulant effect, but major dietary changes—such as a vegetable-rich weight-reducing diet or the use of vitamin K-containing liquid nutritional supplements—can decrease anticoagulation.

See Food Interaction #F-2 for a list of vitamin K-rich foods.

PHENYTOIN AND $\longleftrightarrow$ WARFARIN
OTHER HYDANTOINS

446   824   568

Reaction: Prolongation of prothrombin time with increased risk of hemorrhage.

Suggestion: Monitor prothrombin time closely, and adjust anticoagulant dosage accordingly, both during and following concurrent therapy.

Note: These other hydantoins can react the same way: #824 ethotoin and #824 mephenytoin.

ANTICONVULSANTS $\longleftrightarrow$ CONTRACEPTIVES, ORAL/ESTROGENS

104	322	456	588	404	584	816
150	366	494	746	576	586	860
168	420	530	772			
188	430	532	774			
216	434	552	824			
268	446	558	870			

Reactions: 1. Decreased effectiveness of estrogens and 25-fold increased risk of unplanned pregnancy in women taking oral contraceptives. *Possible* exceptions are contraceptives containing only progestogens: #404 norethindrone (Micronor, Nor-Q.D.) or #576 norgestrel (Ovrette).
2. Breakthrough menopausal symptoms can occur in women on estrogen replacement therapy.

Suggestions: 1. Oral contraceptives should not be relied upon by women taking anticonvulsants.
2. During concurrent anticonvulsant and estrogen replacement therapy, estrogen dosage may have to be increased if breakthrough menopausal symptoms occur.

I-327

PRIMIDONE   ⟷   VALPROIC ACID

456   558

Reactions: 1. Possible primidone toxicity. Toxic effects may include ataxia, confusion, and excessive sedation.
2. Additive CNS depression.

Suggestions: 1. When this combination is unavoidable, advise patients to promptly report any toxic symptoms.
2. See Interaction #I-435.

I-329

ANTICONVULSANTS   ⟷   ANTIPSYCHOTICS

104	322	456	588		174	330	468	768
150	366	494	746		260	370	472	848
168	420	530	772		290	466	758	884
188	430	532	774					
216	434	552	824					
268	446	558	870					

Reactions: 1. High antipsychotic dosage may decrease the anticonvulsant effect.
2. Additive CNS depression.

Suggestions: Monitor seizure control. If increased anticonvulsant dosage becomes necessary, watch for CNS depression. (See Interaction #I-435).

I-331

POTASSIUM CHLORIDE ⟷ POTASSIUM-ELEVATING DRUGS (OTHER)

856

142	422	512
328	424	546
340	508	854

Reaction: Possible hyperkalemia, with muscular weakness to flaccid paralysis and EKG changes ranging from minor sinus bradycardia to ventricular fibrillation.

Suggestions: Monitor electrolytes periodically in patients receiving supplementary potassium.

When possible, substitute potassium-free preparations for those that contain it (such as parenteral potassium penicillins).

Use potassium-sparing diuretics and potassium-containing salt substitutes with caution.

See Food Interaction #F-13 for a list of potassium-rich foods.

I-333

ANTICONVULSANTS ⟷ TRICYCLIC ANTIDEPRESSANTS

104	322	494	746	888
150	366	530	772	
168	420	532	774	
188	430	552	870	
216	434	558		
268	456	588		

Reactions: 1. These drugs are usually mutually antagonistic: Tricyclics can cause seizures and thereby diminish the effect of anticonvulsants; anticonvulsants can diminish the antidepressant effect of tricyclics.
2. Possible additive CNS depression in some individuals.

Suggestions: 1. Monitor seizure control. If the anticonvulsant effect is less than required, reduce tricyclic dosage. (This is preferable to increasing anticonvulsant dosage, which could exacerbate any CNS depression.)
2. See Interaction #I-435.

I-335

ANTIDIABETIC   ⟷   BETA BLOCKERS
AGENTS

176	544	382	476
304	826	392	776

Reactions:
1. Enhanced hypoglycemia, especially with physical exercise.
2. Masking of hypoglycemic warning symptoms: palpitations, nervousness, tachycardia.
3. Possible hypertension during hypoglycemic episodes, often with bradycardia.
4. A mild increase in blood sugar may occur in most diabetics taking beta blockers, and a few will experience a significant increase.

Suggestions: When combined therapy is needed, monitor urine and blood sugar frequently, and advise patients to promptly report any symptoms of hyperglycemia (polyuria, polydipsia, hunger, weight loss, monilial vaginitis, ataxia, drowsiness, lethargy); hypoglycemia (faintness, weakness, palpitations, tachycardia, headache, confusion, ataxia, visual disturbances, sweating). Sweating may be the predominant hypoglycemic symptom in patients taking beta blockers.

Advise patients to keep a candy bar, sugar cube, or other source of simple carbohydrate readily available for hypoglycemic emergencies, and to eat adequate energy-giving foods prior to endurance exercise.

I-337

ANTIDIABETIC   ⟷   CORTICOSTEROIDS,
AGENTS   HIGH
                                      GLUCOCORTICOID

176	544	202
304	826	798

Reaction: Decreased antidiabetic effect via hyperglycemic action of glucocorticoid corticosteroids.

Suggestions: Monitor urine and blood sugar frequently, and adjust antidiabetic dosage accordingly, both during and following concurrent therapy. Anticipate the need for increased antidiabetic dosage during corticosteroid treatment.

Advise patients to promptly report any symptoms of hyperglycemia: polyuria, polydipsia, hunger, weight loss, monilial vaginitis, ataxia, drowsiness, lethargy.

Antidiabetic drug therapy can also cause hypoglycemia. Symptoms may include faintness, weakness, sweating, palpitations, tachycardia, headache, confusion, ataxia, visual disturbances. Advise patients to keep a candy bar, sugar cube, or other source of simple carbohydrate readily available for emergencies.

Note: Applying large quantities of high-potency *topical* corticosteroids may result in significant absorption and systemic activity.

I-339

ANTIDIABETIC AGENTS	⟷	DIURETICS, POTASSIUM-LOSING
176 544		104 276 782
304 826		254 350 882

Reactions: 1. Decreased antidiabetic effect, usually associated with diuretic-induced hypokalemia. Ethacrynic acid (#254) and furosemide (#276) cause this reaction only rarely.
2. When chlorpropamide (#176) and a thiazide diuretic (#882) are used concurrently, increased dilutional hyponatremia may also occur.

Suggestions: Monitor urine and blood sugar and serum potassium during and following concurrent therapy, and adjust dosages accordingly.

Advise patients to promptly report any symptoms of hyperglycemia (polyuria, polydipsia, hunger, weight loss, monilial vaginitis, ataxia, drowsiness, lethargy); hypokalemia (muscular weakness with hypoventilation, diminished GI motility with bloating that can progress to paralytic ileus, polyuria, general weakness, hypotension with dizziness, light-headedness, and faintness); hyponatremia (weakness, confusion, dizziness, anorexia, nausea).

continued

I-339

continued

Preventing hypokalemia appears to minimize any hyperglycemic effect. Hypokalemia may be minimized by:

- Avoiding excessive diuretic doses (eg, greater than 100 mg per day of hydrochlorothiazide).
- Limiting dietary sodium intake.
- Increasing dietary potassium intake. Potassium-rich foods include fresh and dried fruits, fruit juices, fresh vegetables. (Also see Food Interaction #F-13.) Potassium-containing salt substitutes are another useful potassium source.
- Using potassium-sparing diuretics.

Patients developing hypokalemia will require potassium supplementation with liquids, powders, or slow-release tablets.

Note: The following drugs are chemically related to thiazides and will cause the same reaction: #882 chlorthalidone; #882 metolazone; #882 quinethazone.

I-341

ANTIDIABETIC AGENTS	⟷	GLUCAGON
176 544		280
304 826		

Reaction: Possible decreased antidiabetic effect.

Suggestions: Monitor urine and blood sugar frequently, and adjust antidiabetic dosage accordingly, both during and following concurrent therapy.

Advise patients to promptly report any symptoms of hyperglycemia: polyuria, polydipsia, hunger, weight loss, monilial vaginitis, ataxia, drowsiness, lethargy.

Antidiabetic drug therapy can also cause hypoglycemia. Symptoms may include faintness, weakness, sweating, palpitations, tachycardia, headache, confusion, ataxia, visual disturbances. Advise patients to keep a candy bar, sugar cube, or other source of simple carbohydrate readily available for emergencies.

ANTIDIABETIC   ⟷   GUANETHIDINE
AGENTS

| 176 | 544 | | 820 |
| 304 | 826 | | |

Reaction: Possible increased antidiabetic effect.

Suggestions: Monitor urine and blood sugar frequently, and adjust antidiabetic dosage accordingly, both during and following concurrent therapy. Anticipate the need for decreased antidiabetic dosage when starting guanethidine and increased dosage when stopping it.

Advise patients to promptly report any symptoms of hypoglycemia (faintness, weakness, sweating, palpitations, tachycardia, headache, confusion, ataxia, visual disturbances) and hyperglycemia (polyuria, polydipsia, hunger, weight loss, monilial vaginitis, ataxia, drowsiness, lethargy).

Also advise patients to keep a candy bar, sugar cube, or other source of simple carbohydrate readily available for hypoglycemic emergencies.

HYPOGLYCEMICS,   ⟷   PHENYTOIN AND
ORAL   OTHER HYDANTOINS

| 176 | 544 | 826 | 446 | 824 |

Reaction: Possible hyperglycemia, usually occurring after starting or increasing the dosage of phenytoin. Symptoms may include polyuria, polydipsia, hunger, weight loss, monilial vaginitis, ataxia, drowsiness, lethargy.

Suggestions: Monitor urine and blood sugar frequently, both during and following concurrent therapy. Advise patients to promptly report any hyperglycemic symptoms.

If hyperglycemia occurs (as demonstrated by symptoms or urine or blood test) measure serum phenytoin levels, and adjust dosages accordingly.

continued

I-345
continued

Patients on oral hypoglycemics can also experience episodes of hypoglycemia. Symptoms may include faintness, weakness, sweating, palpitations, tachycardia, headache, confusion, ataxia, visual disturbances. Advise patients to keep a candy bar, sugar cube, or other source of simple carbohydrate readily available for emergencies.

Note: These other hydantoins can react the same way: #824 ethotoin and #824 mephenytoin.

I-347

ANTIDIABETIC AGENTS	⟷	MONOAMINE OXIDASE INHIBITORS AND RELATED DRUGS
176 544		274 464 836
304 826		

Reaction: Possible increased hypoglycemic effect.

Suggestions: If this combination is unavoidable, monitor urine and blood sugar both during and for two weeks following concurrent therapy, adjusting antidiabetic dosage accordingly.

Advise patients to promptly report any symptoms of hypoglycemia: faintness, weakness, sweating, palpitations, tachycardia, headache, confusion, ataxia, visual disturbances.

Advise patients to keep a candy bar, sugar cube, or other source of simple carbohydrate readily available for emergencies.

Note: The following drugs are chemically related to MAO inhibitors and can cause the same reaction: #274 furazolidone and #464 procarbazine.

ALCOHOL/   ⟷   THEOPHYLLINE AND
BARBITURATES/   OTHER XANTHINES
BENZODIAZEPINES

108	366	530
168	430	532
188	434	588
216	456	772
268	494	774

902

Reaction: Up to 30% decrease in theophylline effect via increased
theophylline metabolism.

Suggestions: Anticipate possible need for increased theophylline
maintenance dosage when starting barbiturates or benzodiazepines.
Measure serum theophylline levels to verify the need for dosage
adjustment. Theophylline dosage requirements may decrease after
stopping barbiturates or benzodiazepines.

Monitor theophylline levels in patients who regularly consume
alcohol.

Note: These other xanthines may react the same way: #902
aminophylline; #902 oxtriphylline. Dyphylline (#902) is excreted
as unchanged drug in the urine and is unlikely to interact.

ANTIDIABETIC   ⟷   SYMPATHOMIMETICS
AGENTS

176	544
304	826

138	354	592	604
234	378	594	706
248	442	596	876
250	444	598	878
314	480	602	890
318			

Reaction: Possible decreased antidiabetic effect (sympathomimetic
dose-related).

Suggestions: Measure urine and blood sugar frequently during
concurrent therapy. Anticipate possible need for increased
antidiabetic dosage when starting sympathomimetics and decreased
dosage when stopping them.

continued

I-351

continued

Advise patients to promptly report any symptoms of hyperglycemia: polyuria, polydipsia, hunger, weight loss, monilial vaginitis, ataxia, drowsiness, lethargy.

Antidiabetic drug therapy can also cause hypoglycemia. Symptoms may include faintness, weakness, sweating, palpitations, tachycardia, headache, confusion, ataxia, visual disturbances. Advise patients to keep a candy bar, sugar cube, or other source of simple carbohydrate readily available for emergencies.

I-353

ANTIDIABETIC ⟷ THYROID HORMONES
AGENTS

176   544   214
304   826   886

Reaction: Possible decreased antidiabetic effect.

Suggestions: Measure urine and blood sugar frequently during concurrent therapy. Anticipate possible need for increased antidiabetic dosage when starting thyroid hormones and decreased dosage when stopping them.

Advise patients to promptly report any symptoms of hyperglycemia: polyuria, polydipsia, hunger, weight loss, monilial vaginitis, ataxia, drowsiness, lethargy.

Antidiabetic drug therapy can also cause hypoglycemia. Symptoms may include faintness, weakness, sweating, palpitations, tachycardia, headache, confusion, ataxia, visual disturbances. Advise patients to keep a candy bar, sugar cube, or other source of simple carbohydrate readily available for emergencies.

I-355

ANTIDIARRHEALS, ⟷ CLINDAMYCIN
ANTIPERISTALTIC

192   228   752   184

Reaction: Worsening of diarrhea (pseudomembranous colitis) that can be caused by clindamycin, via prolonged contact of clindamycin with the intestinal mucosa.

Suggestions: Avoid this combination. Vancomycin is the recommended treatment for antibiotic-associated pseudomembranous colitis.

ANTIDIARRHEALS,   ⟷   LINCOMYCIN
ANTIPERISTALTIC

192   228   752   324

Reaction: Worsening of diarrhea (pseudomembranous colitis) that can be caused by lincomycin, via prolonged contact of lincomycin with the intestinal mucosa.

Suggestions: Avoid this combination. Vancomycin is the recommended treatment for antibiotic-associated pseudomembranous colitis.

ANTIDOPAMINERGICS ⟷ LEVODOPA

174   370   468   758   320
290   466   472   848

Reaction: Decreased effects of both levodopa and the antidopaminergic.

Suggestion: If this combination is unavoidable, monitor clinical response, and adjust dosage of each drug as indicated.

Note: Levodopa-carbidopa (Sinemet) produces a higher concentration of levodopa with milder, less frequent side effects.

ANTIHYPERTENSIVES   ⟷   ANTIPSYCHOTICS

190	350	438	616	174	330	468	768
218	376	452	760	260	370	472	848
254	382	476	776	290	466	758	884
276	388	504	864				
296	392	508	882				
342	436	546					

Reactions: 1. Additive hypotension, with dizziness, light-headedness, and weakness that may progress to syncope and shock.

continued

I-361
continued

2. If the antihypertensive is a beta blocker (#382, #392, #476, #776), increased beta blocker effect is possible. Symptoms may include bradycardia, hypotension, fatigue, lethargy, arrhythmias, asthmatic symptoms, precipitation or aggravation of Raynaud's disease.
3. Haloperidol (#290) toxicity is more frequent when methyldopa (#376) is given concurrently. Toxic effects may include toxic psychosis with confusion, insomnia, schizophrenia-like symptoms, dystonia, parkinsonism.

Suggestions: 1. Use this combination cautiously. Advise patients to rise slowly from sitting or lying positions. If early symptoms of additive hypotension appear, patients should sit or lie down for a while, and report the occurrence.
2. If a beta blocker is used, watch for evidence of excessive beta blockade, and adjust dosages as necessary.
3. Avoid the haloperidol-methyldopa combination.

I-363
METHYLPHENIDATE ⟷ PHENYTOIN AND OTHER HYDANTOINS

378   446   824

Reaction: Increase in serum phenytoin levels, possibly leading to toxicity. Toxic effects may include ataxia, nystagmus, diplopia.

Suggestion: Advise patients to promptly report any toxic symptoms.

Note: These other hydantoins may react the same way: #824 ethotoin and #824 mephenytoin.

I-365
MONOAMINE OXIDASE INHIBITORS AND RELATED DRUGS ⟷ RESERPINE AND RELATED DRUGS

274   464   836   864

Reaction: Possible excessive stimulation, with marked hypertension, excitement, and hyperpyrexia.

Suggestion: Avoid concurrent or sequential use. Wait 7-14 days or more after stopping MAO inhibitor therapy before starting reserpine. Alternative antihypertensive agents are advised.

Notes: The following drugs are chemically related to MAO inhibitors and can cause the same reaction: #274 furazolidone and #464 procarbazine.

These drugs are chemically related to reserpine and can cause the same reaction: #864 alseroxylon; #864 deserpidine; #864 rauwolfia serpentina (whole root rauwolfia); #864 rescinnamine; #864 syrosingopine.

I-367

ANTIHYPERTENSIVES ⟷ SYMPATHOMIMETICS

190	350	438	616	138	354	592	604
218	376	452	760	234	378	594	706
254	382	476	776	248	442	596	876
276	388	504	820	250	444	598	878
296	392	508	864	314	480	602	890
342	436	546	882	318			

Reactions:

1. Decreased antihypertensive effect. These drugs have a mutually antagonistic effect on blood pressure.
2. Beta blockers (#382, #392, #476, #776) antagonize the bronchodilating effect of sympathomimetics.
3. Combining any beta blocker with any sympathomimetic can sometimes cause paradoxical severe hypertension, with severe headache, visual disturbances, encephalopathy.
4. Paradoxical severe hypertension can also result when guanethidine is combined with a direct-acting sympathomimetic (#'s: 234, 248, 250, 314, 318, 354, 442, 444, 480, 592, 594, 598, 602, 604, 876). See Interaction #I-135 for list of generic names.

Suggestions: Try to avoid this combination. If it cannot be avoided, monitor blood pressure closely.

I-367

continued

Patients taking antihypertensives should seek professional advice before using any nonprescription nose drops or cold remedies, as many contain sympathomimetics. If such products cannot be avoided, they should be used as sparingly as possible.

If a beta blocker must be used in a patient taking a sympathomimetic to relieve bronchospasm, choose one that is relatively cardioselective (has more effect on the heart than the respiratory tract), such as #776 atenolol or #382 metoprolol.

I-369

| ANTI-INFLAMMATORY AGENTS, NONSTEROIDAL | ⟷ | ANTI-INFLAMMATORY AGENTS, NONSTEROIDAL |

(Every drug with number listed below interacts with every other drug in the list.)

112	344	606
300	414	762
302	440	866

Reaction: Possible increased risk of GI hemorrhage.

Suggestion: When two or more of these agents must be used together, advise patients to promptly report any abdominal pain, black or tarry stools, unusual tiredness or weakness.

I-371

| ANTINEOPLASTICS | ⟷ | SMALLPOX AND OTHER LIVE VACCINES |

106	158	352	562	496
130	182	368	764	
134	204	464		
144	238	534		

Reaction: Generalized vaccinia and susceptibility to serious and possibly fatal infections (via immunosuppression).

Suggestions: Do not administer live vaccine to patients receiving antineoplastic chemotherapy (including methotrexate for psoriasis).

If vaccination must be done, discontinue antineoplastic agents 1 week before vaccination, and do not resume them for at least 2 weeks following vaccination.

CAFFEINE   ⟷   ANTIPSYCHOTICS

146

174	330	468	768
260	370	472	848
290	466	758	884

Reactions: 1. Possible caffeinism, especially in psychiatric patients, with nervousness, irritability, headache, rapid breathing, tremulousness, fasciculations, insomnia; and caffeine withdrawal, which closely resembles and can potentiate anxiety neurosis.
2. Caffeine can antagonize some of the beneficial effects of antipsychotic drugs.
3. Possible decreased absorption of the antipsychotic when it is taken with tea or coffee.

Suggestion: Patients taking antipsychotics should avoid excessive caffeine intake.

Note: Common sources of caffeine include coffee, tea, cola and many other soft drinks (such as Mountain Dew, Mello Yello—check labels), chocolate, and many nonprescription drug products.

CAFFEINE   ⟷   CONTRACEPTIVES, ORAL/ESTROGENS

146

404	584	816
576	586	860

Reaction: Decreased caffeine metabolism and possible increased caffeine effects, with nervousness, irritability, headache, rapid breathing, tremulousness, fasciculations, insomnia. Caffeine withdrawal may occur.

Suggestion: Patients taking oral contraceptives or other estrogens should limit intake of coffee and other caffeine sources and should watch for symptoms of caffeinism.

Note: Common sources of caffeine include coffee, tea, cola and many other soft drinks (such as Mountain Dew, Mello Yello—check labels), chocolate, and many nonprescription drug products.

I-377
ASCORBIC ACID   ⟷   ASPIRIN

128   112

Reactions: 1. Doses of aspirin in excess of 600 mg per day for more than 1 week can lower plasma levels of ascorbic acid. Symptoms of ascorbic acid deficiency (scurvy) include bleeding gums, sores on tongue, lethargy, drowsiness, weight loss, myalgia, increased skin pigmentation.

2. Doses of ascorbic acid in excess of 2 gm per day can lower urinary pH, increasing serum salicylate levels. Salicylate toxicity can result. Toxic effects may include tinnitus, dizziness, hearing loss, vomiting, restlessness, delirium, lethargy, hyperpnea, and burning in mouth, throat, abdomen.

Suggestions: When patients on chronic aspirin therapy develop signs of ascorbic acid deficiency, consider using an alternative anti-inflammatory drug (eg, ibuprofen, naproxen), and giving supplemental vitamin C.

If large doses of ascorbic acid are given to patients taking aspirin, watch for evidence of salicylate toxicity.

I-379
ASPIRIN   ⟷   HEPARIN

112   294

Reaction: Increased risk of hemorrhage.

Suggestions: Acetaminophen should usually be used instead of aspirin for analgesia in anticoagulated patients. Other alternatives are salicylates that do not irreversibly impair platelet function. They include #866 magnesium salicylate; #866 sodium salicylate; #866 choline salicylate; #866 salsalate; #866 salicylamide.

BARBITURATES/   ⟷   BETA BLOCKERS
PRIMIDONE

366	456	532	382	476
430	494	588	392	776
434	530	772		

Reaction: Barbiturates may reduce the effect of oral beta blockers.

Suggestions: If response to oral beta blocker is less than desired, consider stopping the barbiturate or increasing beta blocker dosage.

If beta blocker dosage is increased, reduce it when the barbiturate is stopped.

Beta blockers excreted largely as unchanged drug in the urine (eg, #776 atenolol and #392 nadolol) will not be affected.

Note: Primidone (#456) is metabolized to phenobarbital and will cause the same reaction.

BETA BLOCKERS   ⟷   THEOPHYLLINE AND
OTHER XANTHINES

382	476	902
392	776	

Reaction: Beta blocker-induced bronchospasm can antagonize theophylline-induced bronchodilation in patients with pulmonary edema.

Suggestions: Cardioselective beta blockers (#776 atenolol and #382 metoprolol) in low doses are less likely to induce bronchospasm.

Carefully observe patients taking theophylline (or related drugs) for deterioration of pulmonary function when starting any beta blocker.

Measure serum theophylline levels after 1 week of combined therapy.

Notes: Timolol (#776) ophthalmic drops undergo sufficient systemic absorption to produce bronchospasm in some patients.

These other xanthines may react as theophylline does: #902 aminophylline; #902 dyphylline; #902 oxtriphylline.

I-385

BARBITURATES/ $\longleftrightarrow$ CORTICOSTEROIDS
PRIMIDONE

366	456	532
430	494	588
434	530	772

202	266
210	798

Reaction: Decreased corticosteroid effect.

Suggestions: If response to the corticosteroid is less than desired, consider stopping the barbiturate or increasing corticosteroid dosage. If corticosteroid dosage is increased, reduce it when the barbiturate is stopped.

Note: Primidone (#456) is metabolized to phenobarbital and will cause the same reaction.

I-387

BARBITURATES/ $\longleftrightarrow$ DIGITOXIN
PRIMIDONE

366	456	532
430	494	588
434	530	772

222

Reaction: Decreased digitoxin effect.

Suggestions: Avoid barbiturates during digitoxin therapy, or use a different digitalis preparation (eg, digoxin).

Note: Primidone (#456) is metabolized to phenobarbital and will cause the same reaction.

I-389

BARBITURATES/ $\longleftrightarrow$ DOXYCYCLINE
PRIMIDONE

366	456	532
430	494	588
434	530	772

240

Reaction: Decreased doxycycline effect.

Suggestions: If response to doxycycline is less than desired, consider stopping the barbiturate or increasing doxycycline dosage by 50%. If doxycycline dosage is increased, reduce it when the barbiturate is stopped.

Note: Primidone (#456) is metabolized to phenobarbital and will cause the same reaction.

BARBITURATES/ PRIMIDONE	⟷	FOLIC ACID
366 456 532		272
430 494 588		
434 530 772		

Reaction: Folic acid deficiency may result from prolonged barbiturate therapy. Symptoms may include fatigue, pallor, nervousness, irritability, GI disturbances, forgetfulness, and megaloblastic anemia.

Suggestions: Advise patients on long-term barbiturate therapy (or pregnant patients) to report any of the above symptoms. Anemia may also indicate folic acid deficiency. Dietary folic acid replacement (with fresh fruit juice and a fresh, uncooked fruit or vegetable daily) will usually correct the problem.

Note: Primidone (#456) is metabolized to phenobarbital and will cause the same reaction.

BARBITURATES/ PRIMIDONE	⟷	GRISEOFULVIN
366 456 532		288
430 494 588		
434 530 772		

Reaction: Decreased griseofulvin effect.

Suggestion: Avoid barbiturates during griseofulvin therapy.

Note: Primidone (#456) is metabolized to phenobarbital and will cause the same reaction.

I-395

BARBITURATES/   ⟷   PHENYTOIN AND
PRIMIDONE   OTHER HYDANTOINS

366	456	532
430	494	588
434	530	772

446   824

Reactions: 1. In some cases, serum phenytoin levels may decrease, and loss of phenytoin effect (seizure control) may result.
2. In other cases, especially with large doses of barbiturates or pre-existing liver dysfunction, serum phenytoin levels can increase, causing excessive sedation and possible phenytoin toxicity. Toxic effects may include ataxia, nystagmus, diplopia.
3. Sometimes the serum phenytoin level is not affected at all.

Suggestions: Monitor patients continuously for evidence of decreased seizure control or phenytoin toxicity.

Measure serum phenytoin levels approximately 2 weeks after starting and stopping barbiturates, and adjust phenytoin dosage accordingly.

See Interaction #I-435 regarding CNS depression.

Notes: Primidone (#456) is metabolized to phenobarbital and will cause the same reactions.

While this interaction is usually described as Barbiturates-Phenytoin, the other hydantoins (#824 ethotoin and #824 mephenytoin) can probably cause the same reactions.

I-397

BARBITURATES/   ⟷   QUINIDINE/QUININE
PRIMIDONE

366	456	532
430	494	588
434	530	772

862

Reaction: Decreased quinidine effect.

Suggestions: If response to quinidine is less than desired, the barbiturate may be the cause. Anticipate the need to increase quinidine dosage when starting the barbiturate and to reduce dosage when stopping it.

Notes: Quinine (#862) is chemically related to quinidine and will cause the same reaction.

Primidone (#456) is metabolized to phenobarbital and will cause the same reaction.

BARBITURATES/   ⟷   RIFAMPIN
PRIMIDONE

366	456	532	490
430	494	588	
434	530	772	

Reaction: Decreased barbiturate effect.

Suggestion: Monitor clinical response to the barbiturate, and adjust its dosage accordingly, both during and following concurrent therapy.

Note: Primidone (#456) is metabolized to phenobarbital and will cause the same reaction.

DIGOXIN   ⟷   METOCLOPRAMIDE

224   380

Reaction: Metoclopramide increases GI motility and may decrease the absorption of digoxin. This is more likely with slow-dissolving digoxin preparations.

Suggestions: If response to digoxin is less than desired or serum digoxin levels are inadequate, make certain that a recognized, rapid-dissolving digoxin product (eg, Lanoxin) is being used.

If the response remains unsatisfactory, reduce metoclopramide dosage, or discontinue it.

BENZODIAZEPINES   ⟷   LEVODOPA

168	216	774	320
188	268		

Reaction: Possible decreased levodopa antiparkinsonian effect (currently documented only with diazepam).

continued

I-403

continued

Suggestions: If response to levodopa is less than desired, stop the benzodiazepine or increase levodopa dosage.

Note: Levodopa-carbidopa (Sinemet) produces a higher concentration of levodopa with milder, less frequent side effects.

I-405

PROPRANOLOL AND ⟷ CIMETIDINE
OTHER BETA
BLOCKERS

| 382 | 476 | 180 |
| 392 | 776 | |

Reaction: Increased blood levels of propranolol. Beta blockers excreted largely as unchanged drug in the urine (eg, #776 atenolol and #392 nadolol) are less likely to react.

Suggestions: Consider starting with lower beta blocker dosage. Monitor patients for evidence of excessive blockade, especially during the first few days of therapy. Symptoms may include bradycardia, hypotension, fatigue, lethargy, arrhythmias, asthmatic symptoms, precipitation or aggravation of Raynaud's disease.

I-407

BETA BLOCKERS ⟷ CLONIDINE

| 382 | 476 | 190 |
| 392 | 776 | |

Reaction: If clonidine is withdrawn suddenly, increased "rebound" hypertension may occur, possibly leading to hypertensive crisis. Symptoms may include restlessness, tremors, tachycardia, irritability, insomnia, headache, abdominal pain and nausea, increased salivation.

Suggestion: To discontinue clonidine, first gradually taper and stop the beta blocker over a period of at least 1 week. Then reduce clonidine dosage gradually.

BETA BLOCKERS   ⟷   CURARIFORM DRUGS

382   476   512   800   802

392   776

Reaction: Possible prolonged curariform effects—especially respiratory depression, which can progress to apnea.

Suggestions: Try to avoid concurrent or sequential use. If this combination is unavoidable, pay particular attention to maintaining respiratory adequacy.

NITROFURANTOIN   ⟷   PROBENECID

400   458

Reaction: Probenecid reduces renal excretion of nitrofurantoin, significantly decreasing its urinary antibacterial effect.

The resulting increase in serum nitrofurantoin levels can cause polyneuropathies that may be permanent.

Suggestion: Avoid this combination.

NITROFURANTOIN   ⟷   SULFINPYRAZONE

400   524

Reaction: Sulfinpyrazone may reduce renal excretion of nitrofurantoin, significantly decreasing its urinary antibacterial effect.

The resulting increase in serum nitrofurantoin levels can cause polyneuropathies that may be permanent.

Suggestion: Avoid this combination.

I-415

BETA BLOCKERS ⟷ ANTI-INFLAMMATORY AGENTS, NONSTEROIDAL

382	476
392	776

112	344	606
300	414	762
302	440	866

Reaction: Possible decreased antihypertensive effect.

Suggestions: If response to beta blocker is less than desired, consider stopping the anti-inflammatory agent or increasing beta blocker dosage.

I-417

BETA BLOCKERS ⟷ MONOAMINE OXIDASE INHIBITORS AND RELATED DRUGS

382	476
392	776

274	464	836

Reaction: Possible significant hypertension (in theory). The manufacturers warn against using these agents together.

Suggestion: Avoid this combination whenever possible.

Note: The following drugs are chemically related to MAO inhibitors and may cause the same reaction: #274 furazolidone and #464 procarbazine.

I-419

PARA-AMINOBENZOIC ACID ⟷ SULFONAMIDES

116

514	522	872
516	526	

Reaction: Topical or oral use of para-aminobenzoic acid antagonizes the sulfonamide effect.

Suggestion: Avoid this combination.

PENICILLINS   ⟷   TETRACYCLINES

122	424	240	416
152	536	306	880
410	844		
422	846		

Reaction: Tetracyclines may antagonize the bactericidal effect of penicillins.

Suggestions: Avoid combined use unless specifically indicated. If combined therapy is appropriate, begin penicillin first, if possible, and use adequate doses of both antibiotics.

METHOXYFLURANE   ⟷   TETRACYCLINES

372	240	416
	386	880

Reaction: Possible additive nephrotoxicity. (Both agents are nephrotoxic.)

Suggestions: Avoid this combination. Doxycycline (#240) may possibly be used safely.

CALCIUM SALTS, IV   ⟷   DIGITALIS GLYCOSIDES

778	222	224	804

Reaction: Increased digitalis effect, possibly leading to toxicity with arrhythmias.

Suggestions: Try to avoid IV calcium in patients on digitalis drugs.

If IV calcium must be given, infuse low doses slowly. Edetate (EDTA) disodium, which can reverse hypercalcemia, should be readily available.

I-427

CARBAMAZEPINE ↔ PROPOXYPHENE

150   474

Reactions: 1. 66% increase in serum carbamazepine levels and increased carbamazepine effect, possibly leading to toxicity. Toxic effects may include dizziness, light-headedness, ataxia, abdominal pain, nausea, vomiting.
2. Additive CNS depression.

Suggestions: 1. Try to select an alternative analgesic.

    If propoxyphene must be given, measure serum carbamazepine levels after 1 week, and watch for evidence of toxicity. When stopping propoxyphene, watch for decreased serum carbamazepine levels and increased dosage requirements.
2. See Interaction #I-435.

I-429

CARBAMAZEPINE ↔ ERYTHROMYCINS/ TROLEANDOMYCIN

150   252   556   814

Reaction: Increase in serum carbamazepine levels, possibly leading to toxicity. Toxic effects may include dizziness, light-headedness, ataxia, abdominal pain, nausea, vomiting.

Suggestions: Try to select a different antibiotic.

When combined therapy is unavoidable, a 50% reduction of carbamazepine dosage is usually needed. Monitor serum carbamazepine levels both during and following concurrent therapy.

I-431

METHOTREXATE ↔ PROBENECID

368   458

Reaction: Decreased renal excretion of methotrexate, possibly leading to toxicity. Toxic effects may include nausea, vomiting, diarrhea, skin and mouth ulcers, GI bleeding, alopecia, skin rashes, renal and hepatic damage, bone marrow depression leading to septicemia.

Suggestions: When combined therapy is necessary, reduce methotrexate dosage, and advise patients to promptly report any toxic symptoms.

FOLIC ACID   ⟷   SULFASALAZINE
272   522

Reaction: Folate deficiency via malabsorption can occur. Symptoms may include fatigue, pallor, nervousness, irritability, GI disturbances, forgetfulness, and megaloblastic anemia.

Suggestions: Increase dietary folate intake (with fresh fruit juice and a fresh, uncooked fruit or vegetable daily), and give sulfasalazine between meals.

If long-term sulfasalazine therapy is indicated, or if folate deficiency symptoms occur, give 1 mg of oral folic acid daily.

CNS DEPRESSANTS   ⟷   CNS DEPRESSANTS

(Every drug with number listed below interacts with every other drug in the list.)

104	192	268	346	390	466	552	758	848
108	216	270	348	406	468	558	768	864
150	226	282	356	408	472	582	772	868
156	228	284	358	412	474	588	774	870
168	242	290	364	420	492	714	780	884
170	256	292	366	428	494	716	782	888
172	258	298	370	430	530	736	784	
174	260	322	372	434	532	746	790	
188	262	330	376	446	548	752	824	
190	264	338	380	456	550	756	840	

Reaction: Additive CNS depression. Each of these drugs depresses CNS function. Milder symptoms include loss of coordination, ataxia, dizziness, mental clouding. Severe symptoms include respiratory and circulatory failure, with eventual coma and death.

Suggestions: Warn patients of the above symptoms and the additive effects of taking two or more depressants.

Specifically, advise patients against drinking alcohol on days that they take CNS depressants.

continued

I-435

continued

Warn patients that any depressant may impair coordination and driving ability.

Note: Primidone (#456) is metabolized to phenobarbital and will cause the same reaction.

I-437

MEPERIDINE   ↔   MONOAMINE OXIDASE INHIBITORS AND RELATED DRUGS

346   274   464   836

Reactions: Acute reactions have occurred with varying signs and symptoms, including excitation, hyperpyrexia, sweating, rigidity, hypotension, unconsciousness, and respiratory impairment.

Suggestions: Avoid meperidine in patients taking MAO inhibitors. Alternative narcotic analgesics (eg, morphine) should be used—cautiously.

Note: The following drugs are chemically related to MAO inhibitors and can cause the same reactions: #274 furazolidone and #464 procarbazine.

I-439

CNS STIMULANTS   ↔   CNS STIMULANTS

(Every drug with number listed below interacts with every other drug in the list.)

138	250	378	592	604	876
146	274	442	594	706	878
234	314	444	596	770	890
236	318	464	598	786	902
248	354	480	602	836	

Reactions: Excessive, additive CNS stimulation, with agitation, nervousness, excitability, insomnia, ataxia, palpitations, high fever, tremors, slurred speech, rapid pulse and breathing.

Excessive and serious hypertensive episodes can occur, with severe headache, confusion, encephalopathy.

Suggestions: Use the lowest possible dose of any CNS stimulant, and, if at all possible, avoid giving more than one at a time. Advise patients that many nonprescription drug products contain sympathomimetics (including most pills, nose drops, and sprays for coughs, colds, hay fever, asthma, and for weight reduction).

When one of the stimulants is a monoamine oxidase inhibitor or related drug (#274, #464, #836), advise patients to avoid all tyramine-containing foods (see Food Interaction #F-6). Severe reactions are possible.

If acute therapy with a myocardial stimulant is needed, dobutamine (#876) is preferred; it is least likely to cause a hypertensive reaction.

For patients requiring both theophylline (#902) and an adrenergic drug for bronchodilation, the risk of CNS side effects can be minimized by selecting an adrenergic with preferential effects on β_2 receptors (the β_2 receptors are in the bronchial musculature). These include #598 terbutaline; #604 isoetharine; #876 albuterol; #592 metaproterenol.

CNS STIMULANTS   ⟷   PROPOXYPHENE

138	274	444	598	836	474
146	314	464	602	876	
234	318	480	604	878	
236	354	592	706	890	
248	378	594	770	902	
250	442	596	786		

Reaction: Increased CNS stimulation that can progress to convulsive disorder may occur if CNS stimulants are used to treat respiratory depression from propoxyphene overdosage.

Suggestions: Do not use CNS stimulants to treat propoxyphene overdosage. Narcotic antagonists, such as naloxone, are preferred.

CEPHALORIDINE   ⟷   ETHACRYNIC ACID

160   254

Reaction: Increased cephaloridine nephrotoxicity. Symptoms may include hematuria, oliguria, polydipsia, anorexia, nausea, vomiting, weakness, drowsiness, dizziness, dyspnea.

Suggestion: Avoid this combination. Select an alternative cephalosporin.

I-445

CEPHALORIDINE   ⟷   FUROSEMIDE

160   276

Reaction: Increased cephaloridine nephrotoxicity. Symptoms may include hematuria, oliguria, polydipsia, anorexia, nausea, vomiting, weakness, drowsiness, dizziness, dyspnea.

Suggestion: Avoid this combination. Select an alternative cephalosporin.

I-447

CEPHALOSPORINS   ⟷   PROBENECID

160   164   618   458
162   590   788

Reaction: Increased cephalosporin blood levels, with possible increased risk of nephrotoxicity. Nephrotoxic symptoms may include hematuria, oliguria, polydipsia, anorexia, nausea, vomiting, weakness, drowsiness, dizziness, dyspnea.

Suggestion: When high cephalosporin doses must be used with probenecid, monitor patients for evidence of nephrotoxicity.

I-449

CHLORAL   ⟷   FUROSEMIDE
DERIVATIVES/
TRICLOFOS

548   790   276

Reactions: Sweating, flushing, tachycardia, hypertension, and hot flashes have occurred with IV furosemide.

Suggestion: Avoid using chloral derivatives in patients requiring IV furosemide.

Note: Triclofos (#548) is chemically related to chloral derivatives and can cause the same reactions.

CHLORAMPHENICOL ⟷ LINCOMYCIN/
CLINDAMYCIN

166   184   324

Reaction: Possible decreased bactericidal effect.

Suggestion: Avoid this combination.

Note: This interaction is based on theoretical considerations; clinical documentation is not available.

CHLORAMPHENICOL ⟷ PHENYTOIN AND
OTHER HYDANTOINS

166   446   824

Reactions: 1. Increased phenytoin serum levels, possibly leading to toxicity. Toxic effects may include ataxia, nystagmus, diplopia.
2. Possible additive bone marrow depression. Symptoms may include chills, fever, sore throat, mouth sores, unusual bruising or bleeding (such as bleeding gums, blood in urine, unusually heavy menstrual periods, rectal bleeding, black or tarry stools), unusual tiredness or weakness.

Suggestions: 1. Monitor serum phenytoin levels during and following concurrent therapy, and adjust phenytoin dosage accordingly. Advise patients to promptly report any toxic symptoms.
2. Avoid chloramphenicol whenever possible. If it must be used, monitor blood count (though of dubious value), and stop the drug as quickly as possible.

Note: While this interaction is usually described as Chloramphenicol-Phenytoin, the other hydantoins (#824 ethotoin and #824 mephenytoin) can probably cause the same reactions.

I-455

CHLORAMPHENICOL ↔ HYPOGLYCEMICS, ORAL

166   176   544   826

Reactions: 1. Increased hypoglycemic effect.
               2. Possible additive bone marrow depression. Symptoms may include chills, fever, sore throat, mouth sores, unusual bruising or bleeding (such as bleeding gums, blood in urine, unusually heavy menstrual periods, rectal bleeding, black or tarry stools), unusual tiredness or weakness.

Suggestions: Monitor urine and blood sugar frequently, both during and following concurrent therapy, and adjust hypoglycemic dosage accordingly. Anticipate the need for decreased antidiabetic dosage when starting chloramphenicol, and increased dosage when stopping it.

Advise patients to promptly report any symptoms of hypoglycemia: faintness, weakness, sweating, palpitations, tachycardia, headache, confusion, ataxia, visual disturbances. Also advise patients to keep a candy bar, sugar cube, or other source of simple carbohydrate readily available for emergencies.

Avoid chloramphenicol whenever possible. If it must be used, monitor CBC (though of dubious value), and stop the drug as soon as possible.

I-457

METHOTREXATE ↔ SALICYLATES

368   112   866

Reaction: Salicylates inhibit renal excretion of methotrexate; higher serum levels and toxicity can occur. Toxic effects may include nausea, vomiting, diarrhea, skin and mouth ulcers, GI bleeding, alopecia, skin rashes, renal and hepatic damage, bone marrow depression leading to septicemia.

Suggestions: Avoid this combination whenever possible.

If combined therapy is unavoidable, monitor serum methotrexate levels, and adjust methotrexate dosage accordingly.

Advise patients to promptly report any toxic symptoms.

Many nonprescription drug products contain salicylates. Patients should seek professional advice before using any nonprescription drug.

Note: Pepto-Bismol (bismuth subsalicylate) is an unexpected source of significant amounts of salicylate.

I-459

CHLORAMPHENICOL ⟷ MYELOSUPPRESSANTS, INCLUDING RADIATION THERAPY

166

104	226	384	492	590
106	238	386	494	618
124	240	400	510	746
130	254	408	514	756
134	260	414	516	758
144	268	416	522	764
150	274	420	526	772
158	276	430	530	774
160	288	434	532	782
162	290	440	534	788
164	298	456	538	818
168	302	464	552	838
172	322	466	554	848
174	344	468	558	862
182	352	472	562	870
188	366	484	572	872
204	368	488	574	880
208	370	490	588	882
216				

Reaction: Possible additive bone marrow depression. Symptoms may include chills, fever, sore throat, mouth sores, unusual bruising or bleeding (such as bleeding gums, blood in urine, unusually heavy menstrual periods, rectal bleeding, black or tarry stools), unusual tiredness or weakness.

Suggestions: Avoid chloramphenicol whenever possible. If it must be used, monitor CBC (though of dubious value), and stop the drug as soon as possible.

I-461
CHLORAMPHENICOL ⟷ PENICILLINS
166

| | 122 | 410 | 424 | 844 |
| | 152 | 422 | 536 | 846 |

Reaction: Chloramphenicol may interfere with the effect of penicillins.

Suggestion: If this combination is indicated, start the penicillin first, and give it in maximal dosage.

Note: This interaction is based primarily on theoretical considerations. In some infections (eg, typhoid), combination therapy with ampicillin and chloramphenicol is indicated.

I-463
CHOLESTYRAMINE ⟷ DIGITALIS GLYCOSIDES
178

222   224   804

Reaction: Decreased digitalis effect.

Suggestion: Give digitalis more than 2 hours before or 3 hours after cholestyramine.

I-465
CHOLESTYRAMINE ⟷ THYROID HORMONES
178

214   886

Reaction: Decreased thyroid effect via decreased absorption.

Suggestions: Separate doses of these agents by at least 5 hours. Monitor therapeutic response by periodic thyroid function tests.

I-467
CHOLINERGICS ⟷ PROCAINAMIDE
246   580   792

460

Reaction: Antagonistic action on skeletal muscle—for example, in myasthenia gravis. Cholinergics lessen muscle weakness; procainamide increases it.

Suggestion: If possible, avoid this combination in patients with myasthenia gravis.

CLINDAMYCIN $\longleftrightarrow$ CURARIFORM DRUGS

184   512   800   802

Reaction: Possible additive neuromuscular blockade; significant respiratory depression can result.

Suggestions: Pay particular attention to maintaining respiratory adequacy.

The #802 blockers are nondepolarizing, and neostigmine may be useful in treating reactions to them. (Nondepolarizing agents compete with acetylcholine at receptor sites; cholinergic drugs increase acetylcholine concentration, displacing #802 blockers.)

ERYTHROMYCINS $\longleftrightarrow$ LINCOMYCIN/
CLINDAMYCIN

252   814   184   324

Reaction: Possible decreased antibacterial effect of clindamycin or lincomycin.

Suggestion: Avoid this combination.

Note: This interaction is based on theoretical considerations; clinical documentation is not available.

CLOFIBRATE $\longleftrightarrow$ HYPOGLYCEMICS,
ORAL

186   176   544   826

Reaction: Increased hypoglycemic effect. Symptoms may include faintness, weakness, sweating, palpitations, tachycardia, headache, confusion, ataxia, visual disturbances.

Suggestions: Monitor blood sugar frequently, and advise patients to promptly report any hypoglycemic symptoms. Also advise patients to keep a candy bar, sugar cube, or other source of simple carbohydrate readily available for emergencies.

I-475

CLONIDINE   ⟷   LEVODOPA

190   320

Reaction: Decreased levodopa antiparkinsonian effect.

Suggestion: Use an alternative antihypertensive agent for patients taking levodopa.

Note: Levodopa-carbidopa (Sinemet) produces a higher concentration of levodopa with milder, less frequent side effects.

I-477

CLONIDINE   ⟷   TOLAZOLINE

190   542

Reaction: Decreased antihypertensive effect of clonidine.

Suggestion: If tolazoline is needed for vasospastic conditions such as Raynaud's disease, substitute another antihypertensive for clonidine.

I-479

CLONIDINE   ⟷   TRICYCLIC ANTIDEPRESSANTS

190   888

Reactions: 1. Decreased antihypertensive effect of clonidine.
                 2. Additive CNS depression.

Suggestions: 1. Avoid this combination. It usually is simpler to find a substitute for clonidine than for the tricyclic antidepressant.
                 2. See Interaction #I-435.

I-481

COLESTIPOL   ⟷   DIGITALIS GLYCOSIDES

194   222   224   804

Reaction: Decreased digitalis effect due to decreased absorption.

Suggestion: Give digitalis preparation 3 hours before or 3 hours after colestipol.

COLESTIPOL   ⟷   THIAZIDES AND RELATED DRUGS

194   882

Reaction: Decreased thiazide effect due to decreased absorption.

Suggestion: Give thiazide 3 hours before or 3 hours after colestipol.

Note: The following drugs are chemically related to thiazides and can react the same way: #882 chlorthalidone; #882 metolazone; #882 quinethazone.

COLESTIPOL   ⟷   THYROID HORMONES

194   214   886

Reaction: Decreased thyroid hormone effect due to decreased absorption.

Suggestion: Give thyroid hormone 3 hours before or 3 hours after colestipol.

COLESTIPOL   ⟷   WARFARIN

194   568

Reaction: Decreased warfarin effect due to decreased absorption.

Suggestion: Give warfarin 3 hours before or 3 hours after colestipol.

CONTRACEPTIVES, ORAL/ESTROGENS   ⟷   CORTICOSTEROIDS

| 404 | 584 | 816 | | 202 | 266 |
| 576 | 586 | 860 | | 210 | 798 |

Reaction: Possible increased corticosteroid effect.

Suggestion: When combined therapy is needed, advise patients to promptly report any adverse corticosteroid side effects: swelling, weight gain, recurrent or persistent infections, excessive thirst and/or urination, gnawing abdominal pain, unusual tiredness or weakness, bone pain.

I-491

GUANETHIDINE ⟷ LOXAPINE/
MOLINDONE

820   330   768

Reaction: Additive hypotension. Postural hypotension (dizziness, light-headedness, weakness) may progress to syncope. Severe hypotension can progress to seizures and shock.

Suggestion: When this combination is unavoidable, advise patients to lie down immediately, rest, then change position slowly if early symptoms of postural hypotension occur.

I-493

CONTRACEPTIVES, ⟷ TRICYCLIC
ORAL/ESTROGENS   ANTIDEPRESSANTS

404   584   816   888
576   586   860

Reaction: Possible increase in tricyclic toxicity. Symptoms may include anticholinergic effects: possible acute glaucoma, blurred vision, constipation, dry mouth, tachycardia, toxic psychosis (agitation, delirium, disorientation), urinary retention; cardiotoxic effects: serious arrhythmias; other neurologic effects: hyperthermia, ataxia, convulsions.

Suggestion: Advise patients to promptly report any toxic symptoms, so that dosage of one of the drugs may be reduced or stopped.

I-495

CORTICOSTEROIDS ⟷ EPHEDRINE

202   266   248
210   798

Reaction: Possible decreased corticosteroid effect via increased corticosteroid metabolism.

Suggestions: Ephedrine therapy can usually be avoided.

When combined therapy must be used, monitor patients for evidence of decreased corticosteroid effect.

Note: Dexamethasone (#798) is the only corticosteroid for which this interaction has been reported, to date.

CORTICOSTEROIDS   ↔   INDOMETHACIN

202	266	302
210	798	

Reaction: Increased risk of gastric ulceration.

Suggestions: When combined therapy is unavoidable, monitor patients and advise them to promptly report any abdominal pain (especially if related to eating), unusual tiredness or weakness, black or tarry stools.

Note: Applying large quantities of high-potency *topical* corticosteroids may result in significant absorption and systemic activity.

CORTICOSTEROIDS   ↔   POTASSIUM-DEPLETING DRUGS (OTHER)

202	266	104	254	334	782
210	798	120	276	336	832
		152	320	350	834
		154	332	498	882

Reactions: 1. Increased risk of hypokalemia.
                  2. Increased sodium and water retention.

Suggestions: Periodic clinical examination and electrolyte determinations are necessary during combination therapy or when either agent is used alone for long periods.

Advise patients to promptly report any symptoms of potassium depletion (muscular weakness with hypoventilation, diminished GI motility with bloating that can progress to paralytic ileus, polyuria, general weakness, hypotension with dizziness, light-headedness, faintness) and sodium excess (thirst, weight loss, palpitations, hypertension, oliguria, confusion, mental and neuromuscular excitability).

Hypokalemia may be minimized by:

- Adding a potassium-sparing diuretic (eg, spironolactone, triamterene) or substituting one for the potassium-depleting diuretic.
- Limiting dietary sodium intake.

continued

I-499

continued

- Increasing dietary potassium intake. Potassium-rich foods include fresh and dried fruits, fruit juices, fresh vegetables. (Also see Food Interaction #F-13.) Potassium-containing salt substitutes are another useful potassium source.
- Giving potassium supplements.
- Choosing a thiazide diuretic, if possible (eg, hydrochlorothiazide), and prescribing it for alternate-day use.

Note: The following drugs are chemically related to thiazide diuretics and will cause the same reactions: #882 chlorthalidone; #882 metolazone; #882 quinethazone.

I-501

CORTICOSTEROIDS   ⟷   RIFAMPIN

202	266	490
210	798	

Reaction: Decreased corticosteroid effect.

Suggestions: If combined therapy is needed, corticosteroid dosage will probably need to be increased, probably by 100%, to obtain the required effect. Monitor patients for evidence of inadequate corticosteroid effect.

If rifampin is discontinued, anticipate the need to reduce corticosteroid dosage, and monitor patients for evidence of corticosteroid overactivity: swelling, weight gain, recurrent or persistent infections, excessive thirst and/or urination, gnawing abdominal pain, unusual tiredness or weakness, bone pain.

I-503

CORTICOSTEROIDS   ⟷   SALICYLATES

202	266	112 866
210	798	

Reactions:
1. Increased risk of GI ulceration.
2. Reduced serum salicylate concentrations.
3. Possible salicylism when corticosteroids are stopped. Symptoms may include tinnitus, dizziness, hearing loss, vomiting, restlessness, delirium, lethargy, hyperpnea, and burning in mouth, throat, abdomen.

Suggestions: Advise patients to promptly report any abdominal
pain (especially if related to eating), unusual tiredness
or weakness, black or tarry stools, and tinnitus,
hearing loss, or other symptoms of salicylism.

Notes: Applying large quantities of high-potency *topical*
corticosteroids may result in significant absorption and systemic
activity.

Pepto-Bismol (bismuth subsalicylate) is an unexpected source of
significant amounts of salicylate.

I-505

CORTICOSTEROIDS	⟷	SMALLPOX AND OTHER LIVE VACCINES
202 266		496
210 798		

Reaction: Possible generalized vaccinia and susceptibility to serious
and possibly fatal infections (via immunosuppression).

Suggestions: Do not administer live vaccine to patients taking
corticosteroids.

If vaccination must be done, discontinue corticosteroid 3 days
before vaccination, and do not resume it for at least 2 weeks
following vaccination.

This precaution also applies to any corticosteroid used topically
(for EENT or dermatologic conditions).

I-507

CORTICOTROPIN ⟷ POTASSIUM-DEPLETING DRUGS

200	104	210	332	782
	120	254	334	798
	152	266	336	832
	154	276	350	834
	202	320	498	882

Reactions: 1. Increased risk of hypokalemia.
2. Increased sodium and water retention.

continued

I-507
continued

Suggestions: Periodic clinical examination and electrolyte determinations are necessary during combination therapy and also when either agent is used alone for long periods.

Advise patients to report any symptoms of potassium depletion (muscular weakness with hypoventilation, diminished GI motility with bloating that can progress to paralytic ileus, polyuria, general weakness, hypotension with dizziness, light-headedness, faintness) and sodium excess (thirst, weight loss, palpitations, hypertension, oliguria, confusion, mental and neuromuscular excitability).

Hypokalemia may be minimized by:

- Adding a potassium-sparing diuretic (eg, spironolactone, triamterene) or substituting one for the potassium-depleting diuretic.
- Limiting dietary sodium intake.
- Increasing dietary potassium intake. Potassium-rich foods include fresh and dried fruits, fruit juices, fresh vegetables. (Also see Food Interaction #F-13.) Potassium-containing salt substitutes are another useful potassium source.
- Giving potassium supplements.
- Choosing a thiazide diuretic, if possible (eg, hydrochlorothiazide), and prescribing it for alternate-day use.

Note: The following drugs are chemically related to thiazide diuretics and will cause the same reactions: #882 chlorthalidone; #882 metolazone; #882 quinethazone.

I-509
CURARIFORM DRUGS ⟷ DIGITALIS GLYCOSIDES

512   800   802   222   224   804

Reaction: Possible cardiac arrhythmias due to potentiation of digitalis cardiac effects.

Suggestions: If a curariform drug must be used in a digitalized patient, use the lowest possible dosage, and anticipate possible arrhythmias.

CURARIFORM DRUGS ⟷ LIDOCAINE
512 800 802 322

Reaction: Possible increased respiratory depression.

Suggestion: When these agents must be used together, pay particular attention to maintaining respiratory adequacy.

CURARIFORM DRUGS ⟷ LINCOMYCIN
512 800 802 324

Reaction: Possible additive neuromuscular blockade; significant respiratory depression can result.

Suggestions: Pay particular attention to maintaining respiratory adequacy.

The #802 blockers are nondepolarizing, and neostigmine may be useful in treating reactions to them. (Nondepolarizing agents compete with acetylcholine at receptor sites; cholinergic drugs increase acetylcholine concentration, displacing #802 blockers.)

CURARIFORM DRUGS ⟷ LITHIUM
512 800 802 326

Reaction: Additive neuromuscular blockade; respiratory depression can result.

Suggestions: Pay particular attention to maintaining respiratory adequacy.

The #802 blockers are nondepolarizing, and neostigmine may be useful in treating reactions to them. (Nondepolarizing agents compete with acetylcholine at receptor sites; cholinergic drugs increase acetylcholine concentration, displacing #802 blockers.)

I-517

CURARIFORM DRUGS ⟷ MAGNESIUM SULFATE, PARENTERAL

512   800   802   338

Reaction: Additive neuromuscular blockade; respiratory depression can result.

Suggestions: Try to avoid this combination. When it cannot be avoided, pay particular attention to maintaining respiratory adequacy.

Should significant respiratory depression occur, parenteral calcium might be used for treatment. Neostigmine may be useful in treating reactions to the nondepolarizing (#802) blockers. (See Interaction #I-515.)

I-519

CURARIFORM DRUGS ⟷ POLYMYXINS

512   800   802   196   198   450

Reaction: Additive neuromuscular blockade; respiratory depression can result.

Suggestion: Pay particular attention to maintaining respiratory adequacy.

Note: Penicillins and erythromycins have not been reported to cause neuromuscular blockade.

I-521

CURARIFORM DRUGS ⟷ POTASSIUM-DEPLETING DRUGS

512   800   802

104	210	332	782
120	254	334	798
152	266	336	832
154	276	350	834
202	320	498	882

Reaction: Hypokalemia enhances the neuromuscular blocking effect of curariform drugs. The most serious consequence is respiratory depression that can progress to apnea.

Suggestion: Check electrolytes preoperatively. When potassium levels are under 3 mEq/L, anesthesia and surgery should be deferred if possible.

Note: The following drugs are chemically related to thiazide diuretics and will cause the same reaction: #882 chlorthalidone; #882 metolazone; #882 quinethazone.

I-523

CURARIFORM DRUGS ⟷ PROCAINE
512 800 802   462

Reaction: Larger-than-normal doses of procaine, given IV, can cause additive neuromuscular blockade with respiratory depression.

Suggestion: Be alert to this possibility during surgical anesthesia.

I-525

CURARIFORM DRUGS ⟷ QUINIDINE/QUININE
512 800 802   862

Reaction: Additive neuromuscular blockade, especially respiratory depression that can progress to apnea.

Suggestion: If concurrent or sequential use is unavoidable, pay particular attention to maintaining respiratory adequacy.

Note: Quinine (#862) is chemically related to quinidine and will cause the same reaction.

I-527

CURARIFORM DRUGS ⟷ TETRACYCLINES
512 800 802   240 416
                                        386 880

Reaction: Possible additive neuromuscular blockade, especially respiratory depression. An outdated tetracycline product that has deteriorated can cause hypokalemia, leading to further neuromuscular blockade.

continued

I-527
continued

Suggestions: Check electrolytes preoperatively. When potassium levels are under 3 mEq/L, anesthesia and surgery should be deferred if possible.

Advise patients not to use outdated tetracycline prescriptions.

If surgery is necessary, choose an alternative antibiotic, such as penicillin.

I-529
CYCLOSERINE   ⟷   ISONIAZID

206   310

Reaction: Additive CNS toxicity. Toxic effects may include dizziness, drowsiness, muscle twitching, nervousness, convulsions, and psychotic reactions.

Suggestions: Advise patients to promptly report any toxic symptoms. If symptoms occur, the cycloserine should usually be stopped.

I-531
DEXTROMETHORPHAN ⟷ MONOAMINE OXIDASE INHIBITORS AND RELATED DRUGS

212   274   464   836

Reaction: Possible serious CNS excitation or depression. (One death has been reported.)

Suggestions: Avoid this combination.

Advise patients taking MAO inhibitors to seek professional advice before using any nonprescription cough remedies, as many contain dextromethorphan.

Note: The following drugs are chemically related to MAO inhibitors and may cause the same reaction: #274 furazolidone and #464 procarbazine.

DIAZOXIDE   ⟷   PHENYTOIN AND
OTHER HYDANTOINS

218   446   824

Reactions: 1. Decreased phenytoin anticonvulsant effect.
                2. Possible additive hypotension. Postural
                   hypotension (dizziness, light-headedness,
                   weakness) can progress to syncope.

Suggestions: 1. If combined therapy is needed, monitor serum
                   phenytoin levels and clinical response. If
                   anticonvulsant activity decreases significantly,
                   substitute another antihypertensive agent for
                   diazoxide.
                2. Advise patients to lie down immediately, rest, then
                   change position slowly if early symptoms of
                   postural hypotension occur. Also advise patients to
                   promptly report any such symptoms.

Note: While this interaction is usually described as Diazoxide-
Phenytoin, the other hydantoins (#824 ethotoin and #824
mephenytoin) can probably cause the same reactions.

DIAZOXIDE   ⟷   HYDRALAZINE

218   296

Reaction: Additive hypotension. Postural hypotension (dizziness,
light-headedness, weakness) can progress to syncope. Severe
hypotension can progress to seizures and shock.

Suggestions: Advise patients to lie down immediately, rest, then
change position slowly if early symptoms of postural hypotension
occur. Also advise patients to promptly report any such symptoms.

Patients should avoid alcohol while taking these drugs.

I-537

DIGITALIS
GLYCOSIDES

⟷

POTASSIUM-
DEPLETING DRUGS

222   224   804

104	210	320	798
120	254	350	832
152	266	498	834
154	276	782	882
202			

Reaction: Hypokalemia increases the sensitivity of the myocardium to digitalis; cardiotoxicity with serious arrhythmias can result.

Suggestions: Monitor EKG and electrolytes frequently.

Advise patients to promptly report any symptoms of potassium depletion (muscular weakness or cramps, diminished GI motility with bloating that can progress to paralytic ileus, polyuria, general weakness, hypotension with dizziness, light-headedness, faintness) and digitalis toxicity (anorexia, nausea and vomiting, confusion, blurred vision, photophobia, unusual fatigue or weakness, headache, bradycardia or tachycardia, arrhythmias).

See Interaction #I-499 for ways to minimize hypokalemia.

Note: The following drugs are chemically related to thiazide diuretics and will cause the same reaction: #882 chlorthalidone; #882 metolazone; #882 quinethazone.

I-539

DIGITALIS
GLYCOSIDES

⟷

SYMPATHOMIMETICS

222   224   804

138	354	592	604
234	378	594	706
248	442	596	876
250	444	598	878
314	480	602	890
318			

Reaction: Possible additive myocardial effect; arrhythmias.

Suggestions: Avoid this combination.

Advise patients taking digitalis to seek professional advice before using any nonprescription nose drops or cold remedies, as many contain sympathomimetics.

DIGITOXIN   ⟷   RIFAMPIN

222   490

Reaction: Possible decreased digitoxin effect.

Suggestions: Digoxin is preferred in this situation; rifampin's effect on it is minimal.

If digitoxin must be used, monitor clinical effect and increase digitoxin dosage as indicated.

DIGOXIN   ⟷   NEOMYCIN, ORAL

224   396

Reaction: Decreased digoxin effect due to diminished absorption.

Suggestion: Monitor digoxin levels, and increase dosage as needed. Spacing the doses of the two drugs may not prevent this interaction.

METHOTREXATE   ⟷   PHENYLBUTAZONE

368   440

Reaction: Increased response to methotrexate, possibly leading to toxicity. Toxic effects may include nausea, vomiting, diarrhea, skin and mouth ulcers, GI bleeding, alopecia, skin rashes, renal and hepatic damage, bone marrow depression leading to septicemia.

Suggestions: Try to avoid this combination.

When it cannot be avoided, advise patients to promptly report any toxic symptoms.

DIGOXIN   ⟷   SPIRONOLACTONE

224   508

Reaction: Possible increased digoxin effect due to decreased renal excretion. Cardiotoxicity may result.

continued

I-547

continued

Suggestions: Monitor digoxin levels and clinical response, and adjust digoxin dosage accordingly, both during concurrent therapy and after stopping spironolactone.

Notes: Spironolactone is a potassium-sparing diuretic. With potassium-depleting diuretics, digoxin toxicity may result from hypokalemia; but with spironolactone, the mechanism is decreased renal excretion.

Spironolactone may cross-react with the antibodies in some assay procedures, resulting in a false elevation of the measured serum digoxin concentration.

I-549

DIGOXIN	⟷	SULFASALAZINE
224		522

Reaction: Decreased digoxin effect; mechanism uncertain.

Suggestion: Monitor the digoxin levels both during and following concurrent therapy, and adjust digoxin dosage accordingly.

I-551

DISULFIRAM	⟷	PHENYTOIN AND OTHER HYDANTOINS
232		446 824

Reaction: Increase in serum phenytoin levels, possibly leading to toxicity. Toxic effects may include ataxia, nystagmus, diplopia.

Suggestions: If combined therapy is needed, monitor serum phenytoin levels, and adjust dosage as needed, both during concurrent therapy and after stopping disulfiram.

Advise patients to promptly report any toxic symptoms.

Note: While this interaction is usually described as Disulfiram-Phenytoin, the other hydantoins (#824 ethotoin and #824 mephenytoin) can probably cause the same reactions.

I-553

DISULFIRAM   ⟷   ISONIAZID

232   310

Reactions: Psychotic episodes, ataxia.

Suggestion: Avoid this combination.

I-555

DISULFIRAM   ⟷   METRONIDAZOLE

232   384

Reaction: Possible confusion, episodes of psychotic behavior.

Suggestion: Avoid this combination.

I-557

DISULFIRAM   ⟷   PARALDEHYDE

232   420

Reaction: "Disulfiram reaction": dyspnea, dizziness, facial flushing, severe headache, chest pain, blurred vision, thirst, nausea, vomiting.

Suggestion: Do not give disulfiram to any patient who is taking or has recently taken paraldehyde.

I-559

DIURETICS,   ⟷   LITHIUM
POTASSIUM-LOSING

104   276   782   326
254   350   882

Reaction: Increase in serum lithium levels, possibly leading to toxicity. Toxic effects may include dry mouth, weakness, slurred speech, dizziness, abdominal pain, lethargy, anorexia, nausea, vomiting, ataxia, confusion.

Suggestions: If combined therapy is necessary, monitor serum lithium levels, and adjust lithium dosage as indicated. Anticipate lithium dosage reductions of 40-70% when adding thiazide diuretics.

continued

I-559
continued

Advise patients to promptly report any toxic symptoms. In severe toxicity, hemodialysis may be needed. (Lesser measures to try first include diuresis and urinary alkalinization.)

Increased lithium levels appear to be related to diuretic-caused hypokalemia. Therefore, monitor serum electrolytes, and anticipate or treat hypokalemia. See Interaction #I-499 for ways to minimize hypokalemia.

Note: The following drugs are chemically related to thiazide diuretics and can cause the same reaction: #882 chlorthalidone; #882 metolazone; #882 quinethazone.

I-561
ERGOT ALKALOIDS ⟷ SYMPATHOMIMETICS

812	138	354	592	604
	234	378	594	706
	248	442	596	876
	250	444	598	878
	314	480	602	890
	318			

Reaction: Possible additive peripheral vasoconstriction.

Suggestion: Avoid this combination.

I-563
METHENAMINE ⟷ URINARY ALKALINIZERS

360	104	336	726
	332	500	728
	334	722	782

Reaction: Urinary alkalinizers (especially antacids) raise urinary pH; above 5.5, methenamine becomes ineffective.

Suggestion: If antacids or other alkalinizers are required, select an alternative urinary antiseptic or antibiotic.

See Food Interaction #F-11.

ECHOTHIOPHATE   ⟷   PROCAINE

244   462

Reaction: Possible cardiovascular collapse.

Suggestion: Avoid this combination. Substitute another local anesthetic for the procaine.

ECHOTHIOPHATE   ⟷   SUCCINYLCHOLINE

244   512

Reaction: Prolonged, possibly fatal apnea due to potentiation of succinylcholine.

Suggestions: Avoid this combination. If a curare-like drug must be used, choose one other than succinylcholine.

METHENAMINE   ⟷   SULFONAMIDES

360   514   522   872
                            516   526

Reaction: Methenamine acidifies the urine, increasing the possibility of sulfonamide crystalluria.

Suggestion: Discontinue methenamine prophylaxis during sulfonamide therapy.

ANTIPSYCHOTICS   ⟷   EPINEPHRINE

174   330   468   768   250
260   370   472   848
290   466   758   884

Reaction: Severe hypotension can result. Dizziness, light-headedness, and weakness may precede syncope. Seizures and shock may follow.

continued

I-571
continued

Suggestions: Advise patients to avoid sudden changes of position, and to sit or lie down should symptoms occur. Also advise patients to promptly report any symptoms.

Note: Albuterol, metaproterenol, or terbutaline may be desirable substitutes for epinephrine in asthmatic conditions; given orally, they have significantly less cardiovascular activity.

I-573
ANTIARRHYTHMICS ⟷ TRICYCLIC ANTIDEPRESSANTS

230   460   862   888

Reaction: Additive EKG effects (prolonged PR, QRS, and QT intervals) with possible increased cardiotoxic effects such as arrhythmias and cardiac depression.

Suggestions: Try to avoid using the antiarrhythmics with numbers listed above to treat arrhythmias from antidepressant overdosage.

When combined therapy is unavoidable, carefully monitor patients for EKG changes suggestive of toxicity.

I-575
CONTRACEPTIVES, ⟷ FOLIC ACID
ORAL/ESTROGENS

404   584   816   272
576   586   860

Reaction: Possible folic acid deficiency. Symptoms may include fatigue, pallor, nervousness, irritability, GI disturbances, forgetfulness, and megaloblastic anemia.

Suggestions: Advise patients taking oral contraceptives or other estrogens to promptly report any of the above symptoms. Anemia may also indicate folic acid deficiency. Dietary folic acid replacement (with fresh fruit juice and a fresh, uncooked vegetable each day) will usually correct the problem.

HEPATIC ENZYME   ⟷   METHADONE
INDUCERS

150	456	532	356
366	490	588	
430	494	772	
434	530	824	
446			

Reaction: Any of the known hepatic enzyme inducers (carbamazepine, barbiturates, hydantoins, rifampin) can decrease serum methadone levels by increasing the rate of its metabolism. The following symptoms of methadone withdrawal can occur: early—respiratory stimulation, tremors, diarrhea; later—respiratory and circulatory depression, convulsions, hypothermia, pulmonary edema.

Suggestions: Anticipate possible need for increased methadone dosage when adding any hepatic enzyme inducer.

Observe patients for early withdrawal symptoms during the first 1–2 weeks of therapy with a hepatic enzyme inducer. Anticipate the need to reduce methadone dosage to its previous level over the first few weeks after stopping the other drug.

HYDRALAZINE/   ⟷   PYRIDOXINE
ISONIAZID

| 296 | 310 | 482 |

Reaction: During hydralazine or isoniazid therapy, 2–6% of patients will develop a peripheral neuropathy from pyridoxine (vitamin B_6) deficiency. Initial symptoms include numbness and tingling of the feet that can progress up the legs as paresthesias, tenderness, weakness, and other neurological deficits. Reactions are more likely with higher dosages of isoniazid (over 6 mg/kg/day). Malnourished patients are especially at risk.

Suggestions: Give prophylactic supplemental pyridoxine to malnourished patients and those on high-dosage therapy with hydralazine or isoniazid. Monitor all patients for early symptoms of neuropathy; give pyridoxine if any occur.

Alternatively, give prophylactic pyridoxine to all high-risk patients taking isoniazid or hydralazine.

I-581

ERYTHROMYCINS   ⟷   PENICILLINS

252   814

122	424
152	536
410	844
422	846

Reaction: Unpredictably, the effect of either drug may be diminished or enhanced.

Suggestion: It is preferable to use alternative second drugs with either agent.

Note: This interaction is based mainly on theoretical considerations; substantial clinical evidence is lacking.

I-583

ERYTHROMYCINS   ⟷   THEOPHYLLINE AND OTHER XANTHINES

252   814   902

Reaction: Increased xanthine (predominantly theophylline) effect, possibly leading to toxicity. Toxic effects may include GI upset with nausea and vomiting, headache, irritability, dizziness, tremors, insomnia, seizures, tachycardia, cardiac arrhythmias.

Dyphylline is an exception. It does not metabolize to theophylline and does not cause this reaction.

Suggestion: Select an alternative antibiotic whenever possible.

If combined therapy is unavoidable, reduce theophylline dosage by 25%, and measure serum theophylline levels after 2 days.

Note: These other xanthines may react as theophylline does: #902 aminophylline; #902 oxtriphylline.

CONTRACEPTIVES, ⟷ PYRIDOXINE
ORAL/ESTROGENS

404   584   816   482
576   586   860

Reaction: A peripheral neuropathy from pyridoxine (vitamin B_6) deficiency will develop in 2–6% of patients taking oral contraceptives or other estrogens. Initial symptoms include numbness and tingling of the feet that can progress up the legs as paresthesias, tenderness, weakness, and other neurological deficits. Malnourished patients are especially at risk.

Suggestions: Give prophylactic supplemental pyridoxine to malnourished patients. Monitor all others for early symptoms of neuropathy, and give pyridoxine if any occur.

Alternatively, give prophylactic pyridoxine to all high-risk patients on long-term oral contraceptive or estrogen therapy.

FOLIC ACID   ⟷   PHENYTOIN AND
                 OTHER HYDANTOINS

272   446   824

Reactions: **1.** Folic acid deficiency is possible with long-term phenytoin therapy. Symptoms may include fatigue, pallor, nervousness, irritability, GI disturbances, forgetfulness, and megaloblastic anemia.
2. If large doses of folic acid (up to 15 mg/day) are given to correct deficiency, increased phenytoin metabolism is possible, resulting in decreased seizure control.

Suggestions: **1.** Advise patients on long-term phenytoin therapy to promptly report any symptoms of folic acid deficiency. If symptoms occur, a hematological profile is indicated. Anemia may be caused by folic acid deficiency. Oral folic acid (1 mg/day) will usually correct the problem.
2. If clinical effect of phenytoin decreases during folic acid therapy, increase phenytoin dosage.

Note: These other hydantoins may react the same way: #824 ethotoin and #824 mephenytoin.

I-589

LITHIUM   ⟷   SODIUM CHLORIDE

326   502

Reactions: As sodium intake decreases, more lithium is reabsorbed through the kidneys, and lithium toxicity can result. Toxic effects may include dry mouth, weakness, slurred speech, dizziness, abdominal pain, lethargy, anorexia, nausea, vomiting, ataxia, confusion.

As sodium intake increases, more lithium is excreted, and serum lithium may decrease to ineffective levels.

Suggestions: During early therapy with lithium, monitor both serum sodium and serum lithium levels to establish optimal dosage.

Advise patients to maintain a relatively stable sodium intake, and to promptly report any of the following:
- Symptoms of lithium toxicity.
- Starting or stopping a diet.
- Anorexia, vomiting, or diarrhea, which can lead to dehydration with sodium loss.
- Starting or stopping diuretics, which can lead to changes in sodium levels.
- Use of antacids containing sodium (advise patient to check with pharmacist).

See Food Interaction #F-10.

I-591

FUROSEMIDE   ⟷   PHENYTOIN AND OTHER HYDANTOINS

276   446   824

Reaction: Possible decreased furosemide effect.

Suggestion: Monitor patients for inadequate diuresis.

Note: While this interaction is usually described as Furosemide-Phenytoin, the other hydantoins (#824 ethotoin and #824 mephenytoin) can probably cause the same reaction.

LITHIUM   ⟷   PHENOTHIAZINES

326

| 174 | 370 | 468 | 758 |
| 260 | 466 | 472 | 848 |

Reaction: Possible decreased phenothiazine effect.

Suggestions: Monitor clinical response to phenothiazine. If response is inadequate, phenothiazine dosage may need to be increased, and decreased after lithium is stopped.

Note: Concurrent use of lithium and thioridazine (#848) has produced severe neurotoxicity.

METHYLDOPA   ⟷   MONOAMINE OXIDASE INHIBITORS AND RELATED DRUGS

376

274   464   836

Reaction: Decreased methyldopa hypotensive effect.

Suggestion: If control of hypertension diminishes, use an alternative antihypertensive agent during MAO inhibitor therapy.

Note: The following drugs are chemically related to MAO inhibitors and can cause the same reaction: #274 furazolidone and #464 procarbazine.

GUANETHIDINE   ⟷   HALOPERIDOL

820   290

Reaction: Haloperidol antagonizes the antihypertensive effect of guanethidine.

Suggestion: Use a different antihypertensive agent for patients taking haloperidol.

I-599

LITHIUM   ⟷   METHYLDOPA

326   376

Reaction: Increase in serum lithium levels, possibly leading to toxicity. Toxic effects may include dry mouth, weakness, slurred speech, dizziness, abdominal pain, lethargy, anorexia, nausea, vomiting, ataxia, confusion.

Suggestions: Use an alternative antihypertensive agent, if possible.

When these drugs must be given together, monitor serum lithium levels, and advise patients to promptly report any toxic symptoms.

In severe lithium toxicity, hemodialysis may be needed. (Lesser measures to try first include diuresis and urinary alkalinization.)

I-601

GUANETHIDINE   ⟷   METHOTRIMEPRAZINE

820   370

Reaction: Additive hypotension. Postural hypotension (dizziness, light-headedness, weakness) may progress to syncope. Severe hypotension can progress to seizures and shock.

Suggestions: When combined therapy is unavoidable, advise patients to lie down immediately, rest, then change position slowly if early symptoms of postural hypotension occur. Also advise patients that sudden position changes, prolonged standing, hot weather, and alcohol can increase postural hypotension.

I-603

GUANETHIDINE   ⟷   MONOAMINE OXIDASE INHIBITORS AND RELATED DRUGS

820   274   464   836

Reactions: 1. When guanethidine is added to MAO inhibitor therapy, there may be increased sympathetic stimulation and possible severe hypertension.
                      2. When a MAO inhibitor is added to guanethidine therapy, the guanethidine hypotensive effect may be decreased.

Suggestion: Avoid giving guanethidine during and for at least 1 week following the cessation of MAO inhibitor therapy.

Note: The following drugs are chemically related to MAO inhibitors and can cause the same reactions: #274 furazolidone and #464 procarbazine.

GUANETHIDINE   ⟷   PHENOTHIAZINES

820

174	468	758
260	472	848
466		

Reaction: Decreased guanethidine antihypertensive effect.

Suggestions: Use an alternative antihypertensive agent, if possible.

If this combination must be used, monitor blood pressure. If it rises too much, increase guanethidine or decrease phenothiazine dosage.

GUANETHIDINE   ⟷   MINOXIDIL

820   388

Reaction: Additive hypotension that may be severe.

Suggestions: If these agents must be used together, monitor blood pressure closely, and anticipate the need to reduce dosage of either or both agents if excessive hypotension occurs.

ASCORBIC ACID   ⟷   CONTRACEPTIVES, ORAL/ESTROGENS

128

404	584	816
576	586	860

Reactions: High doses of ascorbic acid (1 gm/day) can increase plasma levels of ethinyl estradiol. Withdrawal of ascorbic acid can lead to breakthrough bleeding and possible increased risk of contraceptive failure.

continued

I-609

continued

Suggestions: Intermittent use of ascorbic acid in high doses should be avoided by women taking oral contraceptives containing ethinyl estradiol.

Note: While this interaction has been documented only with ethinyl estradiol, it may be advisable to take the same precautions with any oral contraceptive.

I-611

GUANETHIDINE ⟷ THIOXANTHENES

820 884

Reaction: Decreased guanethidine antihypertensive effect.

Suggestions: Use an alternative antihypertensive agent for patients taking thioxanthenes.

If this combination must be used, monitor blood pressure. If it rises too much, increase guanethidine or decrease thioxanthene dosage.

I-613

GUANETHIDINE ⟷ TRICYCLIC ANTIDEPRESSANTS

820 888

Reaction: Decreased guanethidine antihypertensive effect.

The tricyclic antidepressant doxepin, in doses under 100 mg/day, may not cause this reaction.

Suggestions: It is usually necessary to choose an alternative antihypertensive agent. Satisfactory choices might include diuretics, captopril, or prazosin.

Do not increase guanethidine dosage to try to overcome the antagonizing effect of the tricyclic. Once the tricyclic effect has dissipated, severe hypotensive shock may occur.

DIGOXIN   ⟷   ERYTHROMYCINS/
TETRACYCLINES

224

240   386   814
252   416   880

Reaction: Possible increase in serum digoxin to toxic levels (occurs in about 10% of patients). Toxic effects may include anorexia, nausea and vomiting, confusion, blurred vision, photophobia, unusual fatigue or weakness, headache, bradycardia or tachycardia, arrhythmias.

Suggestions: Advise patients to promptly report any toxic symptoms. If any occur, withhold the next digoxin dose pending further investigation of the cause, and measure serum digoxin levels.

HALOPERIDOL   ⟷   LITHIUM

290   326

Reaction: Increased haloperidol toxicity. Toxic effects may include toxic psychosis with confusion, insomnia, schizophrenia-like symptoms, dystonia, parkinsonism.

Suggestions: Carefully monitor patients for evidence of encephalopathy or extrapyramidal symptoms. If symptoms develop, decreased dosages or change of medication may be necessary.

Note: This combination has been found effective in the treatment of mania.

BETA BLOCKERS   ⟷   CALCIUM BLOCKERS

382   476   910
392   776

Reaction: Possible additive AV blockade and myocardial depression.

Suggestion: This combination, useful in the treatment of hypertension and/or angina pectoris, should be given only under strict, controlled supervision.

I-621

IODINE-CONTAINING ⟷ LITHIUM
COMPOUNDS

312 828   326

Reaction: Additive hypothyroid effect.

Suggestions: Avoid prolonged use of this combination.

Advise patients on lithium therapy to ask their pharmacists about possible iodide content of nonprescription drugs.

I-623

IRON SALTS ⟷ TETRACYCLINES

830   240   416
                        386   880

Reaction: Decreased tetracycline effect due to decreased absorption.

Suggestion: Separate doses of these agents by 3 hours or more.

I-625

ISONIAZID ⟷ RIFAMPIN

310   490

Reaction: Possible additive hepatotoxicity.

Suggestions: Monitor patients for evidence of hepatotoxicity: nonspecific malaise, fatigue, anorexia, right upper quadrant discomfort, jaundice. Patients with previous liver disease and elderly women appear to be at increased risk.

Test liver function every 2 months during combined therapy.

I-627

HEPARIN ⟷ INTRAMUSCULAR
            INJECTIONS

294   306

Reaction: Localized hematomas.

Suggestion: Avoid intramuscular injections during peak heparin administration.

HEPATOTOXINS ⟷ MERCAPTOPURINE

102	188	302	398			352			
104	216	310	400						
108	232	314	404						
112	234	318	414						
124	240	322	416	446	522	558	712	830	878
130	248	354	420	456	526	576	746	860	880
134	250	366	430	486	530	584	772	862	890
138	252	368	434	490	532	586	774	866	
150	268	376	440	494	552	588	816	870	
164	288	378	442	514	554	706	822	872	
168	292	386	444	516	556	708	824	876	

Reaction: Additive hepatotoxicity. Changes may range from mild liver function test abnormalities to frank hepatitis.

Suggestions: Perform liver function tests monthly during therapy with mercaptopurine alone or in combination with any other hepatotoxin. If abnormalities appear, the medications should be stopped, if possible.

ISONIAZID ⟷ PHENYTOIN AND OTHER HYDANTOINS

310	446	824

Reaction: Increased risk of phenytoin toxicity. Toxic effects may include ataxia, nystagmus, diplopia.

Suggestions: Advise patients to promptly report any toxic symptoms. Measure serum phenytoin levels within 1 week after starting isoniazid, and anticipate the need to reduce phenytoin dosage in some patients.

Note: These other hydantoins may react the same way: #824 ethotoin and #824 mephenytoin.

I-633

LEVODOPA   ⟷   PHENYTOIN AND OTHER HYDANTOINS

320   446   824

Reaction: Decreased levodopa effect.

Suggestions: If response to levodopa is less than desired, adjust dosages or substitute another drug for phenytoin.

Notes: These other hydantoins may react the same way: #824 ethotoin and #824 mephenytoin.

Levodopa-carbidopa (Sinemet) produces a higher concentration of levodopa with milder, less frequent side effects.

I-635

LIDOCAINE   ⟷   PHENYTOIN AND OTHER HYDANTOINS

322   446   824

Reaction: Additive cardiac depression with concurrent IV use of both drugs.

Suggestion: Direct-acting sympathomimetics, such as isoproterenol, have been used to reverse bradycardia resulting from this interaction.

Note: These other hydantoins may react the same way: #824 ethotoin and #824 mephenytoin.

I-637

OXYPHENBUTAZONE/   ⟷   PHENYTOIN AND
PHENYLBUTAZONE   OTHER HYDANTOINS

414   440   446   824

Reaction: Increased risk of phenytoin toxicity. Toxic effects may include ataxia, nystagmus, diplopia.

Suggestion: When combined therapy is unavoidable, adjust phenytoin dosage if the serum levels become excessively high or toxic symptoms occur.

Note: These other hydantoins may react the same way: #824 ethotoin and #824 mephenytoin.

I-639

PSEUDOEPHEDRINE ⟷ URINARY
ALKALINIZERS

596

104	336	726
332	500	728
334	722	782

Reaction: Increased tubular reabsorption of pseudoephedrine, possibly leading to toxicity. Toxic effects may include cachexia, hallucinations, personality and behavioral changes, palpitations, dizziness, nervousness, irritability, decreased fatigue.

Suggestions: Limit use of urinary alkalinizers (such as antacids) in patients taking pseudoephedrine. Excessive amounts of alkalinizing foods (dairy products, vegetables, citrus juices, nuts) should also be avoided.

When pseudoephedrine must be continued for prolonged periods, monitor urinary pH, and advise patients to promptly report any toxic symptoms.

I-641

PHENYTOIN AND ⟷ QUINIDINE/QUININE
OTHER HYDANTOINS

446   824   862

Reaction: Possible decreased quinidine effect.

Suggestion: If response to quinidine is less than desired, increase quinidine dosage, or discontinue phenytoin.

Notes: These other hydantoins may react as phenytoin does: #824 ethotoin and #824 mephenytoin.

Quinine (#862) is chemically related to quinidine and may react the same way.

I-643

PHENYTOIN AND ⟷ SULFONAMIDES
OTHER HYDANTOINS

446   824

| 514 | 522 | 872 |
| 516 | 526 | |

Reaction: Increased phenytoin effect, possibly leading to toxicity. Toxic effects may include ataxia, nystagmus, diplopia.

continued

I-643

continued

Suggestion: When combined therapy is unavoidable, adjust phenytoin dosage if serum levels become excessively high or toxic symptoms occur.

Note: These other hydantoins may react the same way: #824 ethotoin and #824 mephenytoin.

I-645

PHENYTOIN AND ⟷ TRICYCLIC
OTHER HYDANTOINS ANTIDEPRESSANTS

446   824   888

Reactions: 1. These drugs are usually mutually antagonistic: Tricyclics can cause seizures and thereby diminish the anticonvulsant effect of phenytoin; phenytoin can diminish the antidepressant effect of tricyclics.
2. In some cases, phenytoin toxicity may also occur. Toxic effects may include ataxia, nystagmus, diplopia.
3. Possible additive CNS depression in some patients.

Suggestions: 1. Monitor seizure control. If the anticonvulsant effect is less than required, reduce tricyclic dosage. (This is preferable to increasing phenytoin dosage, which could exacerbate any CNS depression.)
2. Advise patients to promptly report any symptoms of phenytoin toxicity, so that dosage may be adjusted or an alternative drug used.
3. See Interaction #I-435.

Note: These other hydantoins may react the same way: #824 ethotoin and #824 mephenytoin.

I-647

PHENYTOIN AND ⟷ TRIMETHADIONE
OTHER HYDANTOINS

446   824   552

Reactions: 1. Phenytoin decreases the effectiveness of trimethadione. Increased occurrence of seizures may result.
2. Additive CNS depression.

Suggestions: 1. If seizure control is less than required, increased trimethadione dosage may be necessary until phenytoin is stopped.
2. See Interaction #I-435.

Note: These other hydantoins may react the same way: #824 ethotoin and #824 mephenytoin.

I-649

CIMETIDINE ⟷ PHENYTOIN AND OTHER HYDANTOINS

180 **446 824**

Reaction: Increased plasma levels of phenytoin, possibly leading to toxicity. Toxic effects may include ataxia, nystagmus, diplopia.

Suggestions: Advise patients to report any toxic symptoms.

Measure plasma levels of phenytoin after 5 days of combined therapy, and adjust phenytoin dosage accordingly.

Note: These other hydantoins may react the same way: #824 ethotoin and #824 mephenytoin.

I-651

PHENYTOIN AND ⟷ VITAMIN D OTHER HYDANTOINS

446 824 **566**

Reaction: Decreased vitamin D effect. Bone demineralization with possible osteomalacia or rickets may result. Patients on combined anticonvulsant therapy may be at greater risk.

Suggestions: Patients requiring long-term phenytoin therapy should receive adequate dietary vitamin D and calcium (in fish, milk, and eggs) and sufficient exposure to sunlight.

Patients at high risk should be monitored for decreased serum calcium, increased alkaline phosphatase or bone demineralization, and, if needed, should receive calcium and vitamin D supplementation.

Note: These other hydantoins may react the same way: #824 ethotoin and #824 mephenytoin.

I-653

INFLUENZA VACCINE ⟷ THEOPHYLLINE AND
OTHER XANTHINES

608   902

Reaction: Increase in serum theophylline levels, possibly leading to toxicity. Toxic effects may include GI upset with nausea and vomiting, headache, irritability, dizziness, tremors, insomnia, seizures, tachycardia, cardiac arrhythmias. Toxic effects are more likely in elderly patients.

Suggestions: Theophylline dosage should be reduced by 50% in patients with therapeutic levels who are receiving influenza vaccine. Measure serum theophylline levels 4 to 7 days after vaccination, and readjust theophylline dosage accordingly.

Reduced dosage may be necessary for several weeks following vaccination.

Advise patients to promptly report any toxic symptoms.

Note: These other xanthines may react the same way: #902 aminophylline; #902 oxtriphylline. Dyphylline (#902) is excreted as unchanged drug in the urine and is unlikely to interact.

I-655

HYPOGLYCEMICS,   ⟷   INSULIN
ORAL

176   544   826   304

Reaction: Additive hypoglycemia.

Suggestion: During "crossover" periods (when switching from one agent to the other), monitor blood sugar daily, and adjust dosages accordingly.

I-657

GUANETHIDINE   ⟷   LEVODOPA

820   320

Reaction: Additive hypotension. Postural hypotension (dizziness, light-headedness, weakness) may progress to syncope. Severe hypotension can progress to seizures and shock.

Suggestion: Avoid this combination. Alternative antihypertensive agents are preferred for patients taking levodopa.

Note: Levodopa-carbidopa (Sinemet) produces a higher concentration of levodopa with milder, less frequent side effects.

I-659

HYPOGLYCEMICS, ORAL	⟷	OXYPHENBUTAZONE/ PHENYLBUTAZONE
176 544 826		414 440

Reaction: Increased hypoglycemic effect. Symptoms may include faintness, weakness, sweating, palpitations, tachycardia, headache, confusion, ataxia, visual disturbances.

Suggestions: Monitor urine and blood sugar frequently, and adjust hypoglycemic dosage accordingly, both during and following concurrent therapy.

Advise patients to promptly report any hypoglycemic symptoms. Also advise patients to keep a candy bar, sugar cube, or other source of simple carbohydrate readily available for emergencies.

I-661

LEVODOPA	⟷	METHIONINE
320		362

Reaction: Decreased levodopa effect.

Suggestions: Avoid methionine in patients taking levodopa. Other acidifying agents, such as ammonium chloride or ascorbic acid, should be used instead.

Note: Levodopa-carbidopa (Sinemet) produces a higher concentration of levodopa with milder, less frequent side effects.

I-663

CIMETIDINE   ⟷   THEOPHYLLINE AND OTHER XANTHINES

180   902

Reaction: Increase in serum theophylline levels (via inhibited theophylline metabolism), possibly leading to toxicity. Toxic effects may include GI upset with nausea and vomiting, headache, irritability, dizziness, tremors, insomnia, seizures, tachycardia, cardiac arrhythmias.

Suggestions: When combined therapy is unavoidable, it is imperative to avoid theophylline toxicity. Theophylline dosage should be reduced by at least 50% in patients with therapeutic levels when starting cimetidine. Measure serum theophylline levels after 3 to 4 days of combined therapy, and adjust theophylline dosage accordingly.

Advise patients to report any toxic symptoms.

Note: These other xanthines may react the same way: #902 aminophylline; #902 oxtriphylline. Dyphylline (#902) is excreted as unchanged drug in the urine and is unlikely to interact.

I-665

HYPOGLYCEMICS,   ⟷   PROBENECID
ORAL

176   544   826   458

Reaction: Possible increased hypoglycemic effect (documented only with chlorpropamide, to date). Symptoms may include faintness, weakness, sweating, palpitations, tachycardia, headache, confusion, ataxia, visual disturbances.

Suggestions: Monitor urine and blood sugar frequently, and adjust hypoglycemic dosage accordingly, both during and following concurrent therapy.

Advise patients to promptly report any hypoglycemic symptoms. Also advise patients to keep a candy bar, sugar cube, or other source of simple carbohydrate readily available for emergencies.

HYPOGLYCEMICS,   ⟷   SALICYLATES
ORAL

176   544   826   112   866

Reaction: Possible increased hypoglycemic effect. Symptoms may include faintness, weakness, sweating, palpitations, tachycardia, headache, confusion, ataxia, visual disturbances.

Suggestions: Use caution when giving large doses of salicylates to patients on oral hypoglycemics. Monitor urine and blood sugar frequently, and adjust hypoglycemic dosage accordingly, both during and following concurrent therapy.

Advise patients to promptly report any hypoglycemic symptoms. Also advise patients to keep a candy bar, sugar cube, or other source of simple carbohydrate readily available for emergencies.

Note: Pepto-Bismol (bismuth subsalicylate) is an unexpected source of significant amounts of salicylate.

HYPOGLYCEMICS,   ⟷   SULFONAMIDES
ORAL

176   544   826   514   522   872
                           516   526

Reaction: Possible increased hypoglycemic effect. Symptoms may include faintness, weakness, sweating, palpitations, tachycardia, headache, confusion, ataxia, visual disturbances. The severity of this interaction varies with different combinations of sulfonamides and hypoglycemics.

Suggestions: Monitor urine and blood sugar frequently, and adjust hypoglycemic dosage accordingly, both during and following concurrent therapy.

Advise patients to promptly report any hypoglycemic symptoms. Also advise patients to keep a candy bar, sugar cube, or other source of simple carbohydrate readily available for emergencies.

I-671

INDOMETHACIN   ⟷   PROBENECID

302   458

Reaction: Increased indomethacin effect, possibly leading to toxicity. Toxic effects may include GI symptoms ranging from mild irritation to ulcers and bleeding, headaches, dizziness, somnolence, confusion, blurred vision, tinnitus, deafness, bone marrow depression (with chills, fever, sore throat, weakness), hepatitis.

Suggestions: Anticipate the possible need to reduce indomethacin dosage. Monitor patients for evidence of toxicity.

I-673

LEVODOPA   ⟷   METHYLDOPA

320   376

Reactions:
1. Possible additive hypotension. Postural hypotension (dizziness, light-headedness, weakness) may progress to syncope.
2. Possible decreased levodopa effect.

Suggestions:
1. If symptoms of postural hypotension occur, choose an alternative antihypertensive agent.

   Advise patients to lie down immediately, rest, then change position slowly if early symptoms of postural hypotension occur.

2. If parkinsonism worsens, consider switching to levodopa-carbidopa (Sinemet), which produces a higher concentration of levodopa with milder, less frequent side effects.

I-675

LEVODOPA   ⟷   PAPAVERINE

320   418

Reaction: Possible decreased levodopa effect.

Suggestions: If parkinsonism worsens, discontinue papaverine.

Note: Levodopa-carbidopa (Sinemet) produces a higher concentration of levodopa with milder, less frequent side effects.

LEVODOPA   ⟷   PYRIDOXINE

320   482

Reaction: As little as 10 mg/day of pyridoxine can reverse the levodopa effect.

Suggestions: Levodopa-carbidopa (Sinemet) neutralizes the pyridoxine effect while producing a higher levodopa concentration with milder, less frequent side effects.

Advise patients to check labels on vitamin or mineral preparations, and to avoid taking any with more than 5 mg of pyridoxine per daily dose.

See Food Interaction #F-9 for a list of foods high in pyridoxine.

LEVODOPA   ⟷   RESERPINE AND
                            RELATED DRUGS

320   864

Reaction: Possible decreased levodopa effect.

Suggestion: Alternative antihypertensive agents are preferred for patients taking levodopa.

Notes: Levodopa-carbidopa (Sinemet) produces a higher concentration of levodopa with milder, less frequent side effects.

The following drugs are chemically related to reserpine and will cause the same reaction: #864 alseroxylon; #864 deserpidine; #864 rauwolfia serpentina (whole root rauwolfia); #864 rescinnamine; #864 syrosingopine.

ALCOHOL   ⟷   CAFFEINE

108   146

Reaction: Caffeine does *not* reverse alcohol-induced impairment of performance skills (such as driving). Drinking coffee is not an effective method to "sober-up."

Suggestion: It is important to recognize that drinking coffee does not enable an intoxicated individual to drive an automobile safely.

I-683

LEVODOPA   ⟷   TRICYCLIC
ANTIDEPRESSANTS

320   888

Reaction: Tricyclic antidepressants cause delayed gastric emptying and may decrease the absorption and bioavailability of levodopa.

Suggestions: Give levodopa either 1 hour before or 2 hours after the tricyclic antidepressant.

If response to levodopa is less than desired, dosage adjustment may be necessary.

Note: Levodopa-carbidopa (Sinemet) produces a higher concentration of levodopa with milder, less frequent side effects.

I-685

CIMETIDINE   ⟷   OPIOIDS

180   390   412   840
                            406   752

Reaction: Respiratory depression, confusion, disorientation, and seizures have been reported in a patient with chronic renal failure following the addition of morphine to a regimen of cimetidine and phenytoin.

Suggestions: Carefully observe patients for the above symptoms. Patients with renal failure may require reduced dosage of opioid analgesics.

Notes: The numbers listed above include various opioid analgesics. Current information does not indicate whether all of these agents will produce a similar interaction.

Oxycodone (#412) is not available alone, but is found in such combination products as Percocet-5, Percodan, Tylox.

I-687

AMPHETAMINES   ⟷   TRICYCLIC
ANTIDEPRESSANTS

138   706   888

Reaction: Possible increased CNS stimulation.

Suggestions: This combination can usually be avoided. When it must be used, consider smaller doses of amphetamine, and monitor patients for excessive stimulation.

DIGOXIN   ⟷   METHYLDOPA

224   376

Reactions: Sinus bradycardia, "sick-sinus" syndrome, dizziness, light-headedness, forgetfulness, confusion, possibly progressing to syncope. These reactions are most likely in elderly patients.

Suggestions: Monitor patients for bradycardia, and advise them to report any toxic symptoms.

ALCOHOL   ⟷   CEFAMANDOLE/
                                     MOXALACTAM

108   590   618

Reaction: Possible disulfiram-like reaction: dyspnea, dizziness, facial flushing, severe headache.

Suggestion: Advise patients taking cefamandole or moxalactam to avoid all alcohol, including alcohol-containing medications. Exposure to alcohol-based paints or cosmetics may also cause a reaction in susceptible individuals.

ALLOPURINOL   ⟷   AMPICILLIN/
                                       BACAMPICILLIN

110   122

Reaction: Increased incidence of "ampicillin rash" in patients taking allopurinol (22% vs. 2%).

Suggestion: Because of this possibility, it may be appropriate to select alternative antibiotics for patients taking allopurinol.

I-695

BENZODIAZEPINES ⟷ CIMETIDINE

168   216   774   180
188   268

Reaction: Increased plasma levels of benzodiazepine, with resultant increased sedation and other symptoms of CNS depression, such as loss of coordination, ataxia, dizziness, mental clouding. Symptoms may progress to respiratory and circulatory failure.

Exceptions: Lorazepam (#774) and oxazepam (#774) do not interact this way.

Suggestions: If a benzodiazepine is required during cimetidine therapy, use lorazepam or oxazepam, if possible.

When other benzodiazepines must be used, advise patients against driving or operating any hazardous machinery. Also advise patients to promptly report any sedation or other symptoms of CNS depression. If symptoms occur, choose a different benzodiazepine or reduce dosage.

I-697

BENZODIAZEPINES ⟷ RIFAMPIN

168   216   774   490
188   268

Reaction: Decreased benzodiazepine effect via increased benzodiazepine metabolism.

Suggestions: Monitor benzodiazepine effect; if less than desired, rifampin could be the cause. If necessary, increase benzodiazepine dosage.

Note: Lorazepam (#774) and oxazepam (#774) are less likely to be affected by rifampin.

I-699

ANTACIDS (ALL) ⟷ CIMETIDINE

332   500   726   180
334   722   728
336

Reaction: Decreased oral absorption of cimetidine.

Suggestion: Separate antacid and cimetidine doses by at least 1 hour.

DISOPYRAMIDE $\longleftrightarrow$ RIFAMPIN/
PHENYTOIN AND
OTHER HYDANTOINS

230   446   490   824

Reaction: Decreased disopyramide effect via increased disopyramide metabolism.

Suggestions: Measure plasma levels of disopyramide after 1 week of combined therapy, and adjust disopyramide dosage accordingly. If rifampin or phenytoin is stopped, decreased disopyramide dosage may be necessary.

Note: The other hydantoins (#824 ethotoin and #824 mephenytoin) may react as phenytoin does.

ANTI-INFLAMMATORY $\longleftrightarrow$ FUROSEMIDE/
AGENTS,   THIAZIDES AND
NONSTEROIDAL   RELATED DRUGS

112	344	606	276	882
300	414	762		
302	440	866		

Reaction: Decreased diuretic and antihypertensive effects of furosemide or thiazides.

Suggestions: Monitor patients for inadequate antihypertensive or diuretic effect. Reduce or discontinue anti-inflammatory dosage, as indicated. If that is not feasible, increase diuretic dosage, as needed.

Note: The following drugs are chemically related to thiazides and can cause the same reaction: #882 chlorthalidone; #882 metolazone; #882 quinethazone.

I-705

ANTIHYPERTENSIVES ⟷ MONOAMINE OXIDASE INHIBITORS AND RELATED DRUGS

218	342	438	546	274	464	836
254	350	452	616			
276	388	504	760			
296	436	508	882			

Reaction: Increased risk of postural hypotension, with dizziness, light-headedness, weakness.

Suggestions: Try to avoid this combination.

If it cannot be avoided, advise patient to lie down immediately, rest, then change position slowly if early symptoms of postural hypotension occur. Change of antihypertensive medication or dosage may become necessary.

Note: The following drugs are chemically related to MAO inhibitors and can cause the same reactions: #274 furazolidone and #464 procarbazine.

I-707

LEVODOPA ⟷ MONOAMINE OXIDASE INHIBITORS AND RELATED DRUGS

320   274   464   836

Reaction: Possible severe hypertensive episodes. (Levodopa increases dopamine levels; MAO inhibitors potentiate dopamine stimulation.) Hyperpyrexia, severe headache, visual disturbances, encephalopathy may result.

Suggestions: Try to avoid this combination.

When it cannot be avoided, and symptoms occur, hypertensive episodes can be treated with phentolamine.

Notes: The use of carbidopa-levodopa (Sinemet) may prevent hypertensive reactions.

The following drugs are chemically related to MAO inhibitors and can cause the same reactions: #274 furazolidone and #464 procarbazine.

I-709

CONTRACEPTIVES, ⟷ TROLEANDOMYCIN
ORAL/ESTROGENS

404	584	816	556
576	586	860	

Reaction: Increased risk of cholestatic jaundice.

Suggestion: Avoid this combination. Select an alternative antibiotic for women taking oral contraceptives or other estrogens. See also Interaction #I-107.

I-711

PHENYL- ⟷ INDOMETHACIN
PROPANOLAMINE

444   302

Reaction: Possible increased blood pressure and headache.

Suggestion: Avoid this combination.

I-713

BETA BLOCKERS ⟷ PRAZOSIN

382	476	452
392	776	

Reaction: Increased severity and duration of the "first-dose" postural hypotension caused by prazosin. Dizziness, light-headedness, and weakness can progress to syncope. The usual compensatory tachycardia is blocked by beta blockers.

Suggestions: Standard techniques to reduce the prazosin "first-dose" response include:
- Using the smallest possible initial dose of prazosin (1 mg) and giving the first dose at bedtime.
- Withholding beta blockers on the day before the first prazosin dose.

I-715

DIURETICS   ⟷   PRAZOSIN

104   350   782   452
254   614   882
276

Reaction: In patients taking diuretics, the first dose of prazosin can be followed (within 3 hours) by marked hypotension, with dizziness, light-headedness, and weakness that can progress to syncope. The cause is sodium and/or volume depletion.

Suggestions: Use the smallest possible initial dose of prazosin (1 mg), and give the first dose at bedtime.

Withhold diuretics for 1–2 days before the first prazosin dose.

Advise patients to drink adequate fluids before the first prazosin dose, and to lie down quickly if symptoms of hypotension occur.

I-717

PROCAINAMIDE   ⟷   URINARY ALKALINIZERS

460   104   336   726
                332   500   728
                334   722   782

Reaction: Alkalinization of the urine increases procainamide renal reabsorption, possibly leading to toxicity. Toxic effects may include hypotension via peripheral vasodilation, heart block, ventricular fibrillation.

Suggestions: Patients on urinary alkalinizers (such as antacids) or alkalinizing diets (high in dairy products, vegetables, citrus juices, nuts) may require reduction of procainamide dosage. Monitor patients closely for evidence of toxicity when adding any urinary alkalinizer.

I-719

QUINIDINE/QUININE   ⟷   RIFAMPIN

862   490

Reaction: Increased metabolism and decreased plasma levels of quinidine, with loss of therapeutic effect. Oral quinidine is affected more than IV quinidine.

Suggestions: Measure plasma levels of quinidine within 7 days after starting rifampin, and adjust quinidine dosage accordingly. More than twice the original dosage may be necessary for oral quinidine. When stopping rifampin, anticipate the need to reduce quinidine dosage.

Note: Quinine (#862) is chemically related to quinidine and may react the same way.

I-721

TRICYCLIC   ⟷   FENFLURAMINE
ANTIDEPRESSANTS

888   262

Reaction: Increased fenfluramine sedative and depressant effects.

Suggestion: This combination can nearly always be avoided.

I-723

ALLOPURINOL   ⟷   VIDARABINE

110   610

Reaction: Increased vidarabine neurotoxicity (tremors and impaired mentation).

Suggestions: Monitor patients closely for evidence of toxicity. Anticipate the possible need to reduce vidarabine dosage.

I-725

VITAMIN A   ⟷   TETRACYCLINES

612   240   416
                                 386   880

Reaction: Possible increased risk of benign intracranial hypertension (pseudotumor cerebri). Symptoms may include throbbing headache, visual disturbances, papilledema, nausea, vomiting.

Suggestions: Supplemental vitamin A should generally be avoided by patients on long-term tetracycline therapy (such as for acne).

When this combination must be used, advise patients to stop both drugs and seek medical advice if headache develops.

I-727
CAFFEINE   ⟷   CIMETIDINE

146   180

Reaction: Decreased caffeine metabolism and possible increased caffeine effects. Symptoms may include nervousness, irritability, headache, rapid breathing, tremulousness, fasciculations, insomnia, and caffeine withdrawal.

Suggestions: For most patients taking cimetidine, the condition being treated (eg, peptic ulcer) contraindicates caffeine use. Therefore, caffeine should probably be avoided.

Patients who do use caffeine should moderate their drinking of coffee or other caffeine beverages and should watch for symptoms of caffeinism.

Common sources of caffeine include coffee, tea, cola and many other soft drinks (such as Mountain Dew, Mello Yello—check labels), chocolate, and many nonprescription drug products.

I-729
COUMARIN   ⟷   INFLUENZA VACCINE
ANTICOAGULANTS

140   568   742   608

Reaction: Increased anticoagulant effect; serious internal bleeding can occur.

Suggestions: Avoid giving influenza vaccine, if possible, to patients taking coumarins.

If vaccination must be done, monitor prothrombin time carefully, and reduce anticoagulant dosage if undue prolongation of prothrombin time occurs.

Advise patients to promptly report any unusual bruising or bleeding (such as bleeding gums, blood in urine, unusually heavy menstrual periods, rectal bleeding, black or tarry stools).

Note: Only one case has been reported, to date, but the reaction was severe enough to warrant concern over this combination.

ANTI-INFLAMMATORY ⟷ LITHIUM
AGENTS,
NONSTEROIDAL

112	344	606		326
300	414	762		
302	440	866		

Reaction: Reduced renal clearance of lithium, leading to increased lithium levels and possible toxicity. Toxic effects may include dry mouth, weakness, slurred speech, dizziness, abdominal pain, lethargy, anorexia, nausea, vomiting, ataxia, confusion. This interaction has been documented only with indomethacin, but may be expected with any of the nonsteroidal anti-inflammatory agents.

Suggestions: When these drugs must be taken together for more than a few days, monitor serum lithium levels. Reduce lithium dosage if blood levels are excessive or toxic symptoms occur. Increased lithium dosage may be necessary when the anti-inflammatory agent is stopped.

RIFAMPIN ⟷ TRICYCLIC
ANTIDEPRESSANTS

490   888

Reaction: Possible decreased antidepressant effect via increased tricyclic metabolism.

Suggestions: Patients taking rifampin may require titration to higher than usual doses of the tricyclic antidepressant to obtain the desired effect. After the rifampin is stopped, hepatic metabolism will slowly return to normal, and reduced tricyclic dosage may be necessary after several weeks.

I-735

ANTACIDS   ⟷   ANTICHOLINERGICS

332	500	726	132	226	408	736
334	722	728	136	284	470	738
336			172	312	492	
			220	374	550	

Reaction: Antacids can decrease the absorption and effectiveness of oral anticholinergics.

Suggestion: Separate antacid and anticholinergic doses by at least 1 hour.

Avoid using any anticholinergic drug in patients with glaucoma.

I-737

ANTACIDS   ⟷   NITROFURANTOIN
CONTAINING
MAGNESIUM
TRISILICATE

728   400

Reaction: Magnesium trisilicate antacids reduce the absorption of oral nitrofurantoin.

Suggestion: Avoid simultaneous administration of these two agents.

I-739

CAPTOPRIL   ⟷   DIURETICS/DRUGS
THAT ELEVATE
SERUM POTASSIUM

616	104	328	424	614	882
	142	340	508	782	
	254	350	512	854	
	276	422	546	856	

Reactions: 1. Possible marked hypotension within 3 hours following the initial dose of captopril in patients on any diuretics (#104, #254, #276, #350, #508, #546, #614, #782, #882).
            2. Possible excessive increase in serum potassium in patients on any drugs that elevate serum potassium (#'s: 142, 328, 340, 422, 424, 508, 512, 546, 614, 854, 856).

Suggestions: 1. Use the smallest possible initial dose of captopril, and give the first dose at bedtime. Withhold diuretics for 1–2 days before the first captopril dose. Advise patients to drink adequate fluids before the first captopril dose, and to lie down quickly if symptoms of hypotension (dizziness, light-headedness, weakness) occur.
2. Monitor serum potassium periodically during combined therapy. Potassium excess may result in muscular weakness to flaccid paralysis and EKG changes ranging from minor sinus bradycardia to ventricular fibrillation.

I-741

DIGOXIN ⟷ DRUGS THAT INHIBIT GI MOTILITY

224

132	260	374	474
136	264	390	492
172	284	406	550
192	312	408	736
220	346	412	738
226	356	428	752
228	370	470	840

Reaction: Decreased GI motility can result in increased digoxin absorption and effect, possibly leading to toxicity. Toxic effects may include anorexia, nausea and vomiting, confusion, blurred vision, photophobia, unusual fatigue or weakness, headache, bradycardia or tachycardia, arrhythmias.

Inhibitors of GI motility include anticholinergics, narcotic analgesics, and antiperistaltic antidiarrheals.

Suggestions: When this combination must be given for prolonged periods, monitor serum digoxin levels and watch for evidence of increased digoxin effect.

Notes: Use of a rapid-dissolving digoxin preparation (such as Lanoxin) diminishes the importance of this reaction.

Avoid using any anticholinergic drug (#'s: 132, 136, 172, 220, 226, 260, 284, 312, 374, 408, 470, 492, 550, 736, 738) in patients with glaucoma.

I-743

CIMETIDINE   ⟷   SUCRALFATE

180   620

Reaction: Decreased activity of sucralfate, which requires hydrolysis by stomach acid for its action.

Suggestion: Combined therapy is not recommended.

F-1

FOODS   ⟷   DRUGS WITH INCREASED BIOAVAILABILITY

150   400
216   446

Reaction: Foods increase the absorption of carbamazepine, diazepam, nitrofurantoin, and phenytoin.

Suggestions: Advise patients to take these drugs with food, as consistently as possible. However, the drug dose should be taken even if a meal is skipped.

F-2

FOODS   ⟷   ANTICOAGULANTS, ORAL

140   742
568   744

Reaction: Foods rich in vitamin K antagonize the effect of oral anticoagulants.

Suggestion: Advise patients taking oral anticoagulants to maintain a consistent level of dietary vitamin K intake; to avoid extremes.

Vitamin K-rich foods include leafy green vegetables (asparagus, broccoli, Brussels sprouts, cabbage, kale, lettuce, peas, spinach, turnip greens, watercress), liver, green tea.

See Interaction #I-321.

FOODS   ↔   ANTIHYPERTENSIVE
AGENTS

190	342	436	760
218	350	452	820
254	376	504	864
276	388	546	

Reaction: Natural licorice contains a corticosteroid-type pressor substance (carbenoxolone), which can interfere with the effect of antihypertensive drugs.

Suggestion: Advise patients on antihypertensive therapy to eat no more than an occasional piece of natural licorice.

FOODS   ↔   ISONIAZID

310

Reactions:
1. Isoniazid increases histamine levels by decreasing histamine metabolism. When this effect is further enhanced by foods high in histamine, toxicity can result. Toxic effects may include severe headache, erythema, redness of face. Foods highest in histamine are fish (such as tuna, sardines, skipjack) that have started to spoil—even before any change in taste is detectable.
2. All foods reduce absorption of isoniazid.
3. Isoniazid acts like a monoamine oxidase inhibitor in some cases.

Suggestions:
1. Advise patients taking isoniazid to eat only fish that has been safely stored. Also advise them of the symptoms of histamine toxicity. Should symptoms develop, antihistamines theoretically may reduce or shorten the reaction.
2. Give isoniazid with a full glass of water 1 hour before or 2 hours after meals. But it is better for an occasional dose to be taken with food than to be skipped altogether.
3. See Food Interaction #F-6.

F-5

FOODS   ⟷   ANTIBACTERIALS

122	324	424	814
152	410	490	844
252	422	536	846

Reaction: Foods reduce oral absorption of the following antibacterials: lincomycin and clindamycin, rifampin, most erythromycins (exceptions: erythromycin estolate and enteric-coated erythromycins), and most penicillins (exceptions: amoxicillin, bacampicillin, hetacillin).

Suggestions: Give the antibacterial 1 hour before or 2 hours after meals, with a full 8-ounce glass of water. But it is better for an occasional dose to be taken with food than to be skipped altogether.

Note: Although the effect of acidic juices on penicillin absorption is unclear, it seems reasonable to allow 1 hour to elapse between penicillin doses and drinking fruit juices or other acidic beverages (eg, colas).

F-6

FOODS   ⟷   MONOAMINE OXIDASE INHIBITORS AND RELATED DRUGS

274   464   836

Reaction: When tyramine-containing foods are taken during MAO inhibitor therapy, serious acute hypertension can occur, with possible severe headache, confusion, and somnolence. Brain hemorrhage and death may follow.

Suggestion: Advise patients taking any drug with MAO inhibitor activity to *strictly avoid* foods high in tyramine. The principal foods to avoid include:

avocados	cola beverages	sauerkraut
baked potatoes	fermented products	sausage
bananas	fish	sour cream
bean pods	liver	soy sauce
canned figs	meat tenderizers	wines
cheese	pepperoni	yeast preparations
chicken livers	pickled herring	yogurt
chocolate	raspberries	
coffee	salami	

Note: The following drugs are chemically related to MAO inhibitors and can cause the same reaction: #274 furazolidone and #464 procarbazine.

FOODS　　　　　↔　　　　　GRIEOFULVIN

GRISEOFULVIN

288

Reaction: Foods (particularly fatty foods) increase absorption of griseofulvin.

Suggestions: Advise patients to take griseofulvin with meals. However, the drug dose should be taken even if a meal is skipped.

FOODS　　　　　↔　　　　　BETA BLOCKERS/
HYDRALAZINE/
SPIRONOLACTONE/
THIAZIDES AND
RELATED DRUGS

296	476	776
382	508	882
392		

Reactions:　1. Any of the above medications reaches significantly higher serum levels when taken with foods.
2. Natural licorice contains a corticosteroid-type pressor substance (carbenoxolone), which can interfere with the antihypertensive effect of these drugs.

Suggestions:　1. Advise patients to take these drugs in as consistent a manner as possible, either 1 hour before or 2 hours after any food. The drug dose should be taken even if a meal is skipped.
2. Advise patients taking any of these drugs for antihypertensive therapy to eat no more than an occasional piece of natural licorice.

Note: The following drugs are chemically related to thiazides and can cause the same reaction: #882 chlorthalidone; #882 metolazone; #882 quinethazone.

F-9
FOODS   ⟷   LEVODOPA

320

Reactions: High-protein diets (high in meat and dairy products) decrease levodopa absorption and effect.

As little as 10 mg/day of pyridoxine (vitamin B_6) reverses the antiparkinsonian effects of levodopa.

Suggestions: Advise patients taking levodopa to avoid excessive protein intake, and to take levodopa 1 hour before or 2 hours after meals.

See Interaction #I-677.

Foods high in pyridoxine include:

avocados	peas
beans	pork
bacon	sweet potatoes
beef liver	tuna
dried yeast	vitamin preparations with B_6
dry skim milk	(advise patient to read labels)
oatmeal	

F-10
FOODS   ⟷   LITHIUM

326

Reaction: Serum lithium levels may vary in inverse proportion to sodium intake.

Suggestions: Advise patients taking lithium to maintain salt-balanced diets, and to promptly report significant variations in diet. Measure serum lithium levels at times of dietary change.

A very low-salt diet can cause lithium toxicity (with dry mouth, weakness, slurred speech, dizziness, abdominal pain, lethargy, anorexia, nausea, vomiting, ataxia, confusion), while a high salt intake can lead to therapeutic failure.

Check sodium content of all other medications the patient may be taking.

See Interaction #I-589.

FOODS   ⟷   METHENAMINE

360

Reaction: Methenamine is inactive at a urinary pH greater than 5.5.

Suggestions: If the prescribed medication combines methenamine with one of its acidifying salts (eg, Hiprex, Urex, Mandelamine, Hexalet), but urinary pH remains above 5.5, dietary measures may help. Advise patients to:

Favor acidifying foods: bread, bacon, corn, lentils, meat, fish, fowl, cranberries, plums, prunes.

Minimize or avoid alkalinizing foods: milk and other dairy products, vegetables, almonds, chestnuts, coconuts, citrus juices.

FOODS/SMOKING   ⟷   THEOPHYLLINE AND OTHER XANTHINES

902

Reactions: Theophylline effect is decreased (via increased metabolism) by a high-protein/low-carbohydrate diet; charcoal-broiled beef; smoking of cigarettes or marijuana.

Theophylline effect is increased (via decreased metabolism) by a low-carbohydrate diet or by caffeine. Toxicity can result, with CNS stimulation, GI upset.

Suggestions: Theophylline should be taken with foods to avoid GI upsets, but dietary extremes of proteins or carbohydrates should be avoided.

To avoid significant decreases in theophylline effect, patients should reduce cigarette or marijuana smoking as much as possible, and minimize eating of charcoal-broiled beef. (Even after smoking has been stopped, it may be months before theophylline metabolism returns to normal.)

To avoid possible xanthine toxicity, patients should avoid large amounts of caffeine, found in coffee, tea, cola beverages, chocolate, cocoa, and many nonprescription drug products.

Note: These other xanthines may react the same way: #902 aminophylline; #902 oxtriphylline. Dyphylline (#902) is excreted as unchanged drug in the urine and is unlikely to be affected by foods or smoking.

F-13
FOODS　　　　⟷　　　　POTASSIUM CHLORIDE
856

Reaction: Hyperkalemia may result when supplemental potassium therapy is combined with a diet rich in potassium. Potassium-rich foods include citrus fruits and juices, figs, raisins, bananas, prunes, potatoes, sweet potatoes, winter squash, cantaloupe.

Suggestions: In general, patients taking potassium supplements can eat normal amounts of potassium-containing foods. The risk of hyperkalemia is greatest in patients with reduced renal function.

Monitor serum potassium and clinical symptoms to avoid serious hyperkalemia. Early symptoms prior to serious cardiac arrhythmias are few, but may include GI effects such as cramps, diarrhea, distension.

See Interaction #I-331 regarding potassium-elevating drugs.

F-14
FOODS　　　　⟷　　　　QUINIDINE/QUININE
862

Reaction: Urinary alkalinization may increase quinidine reabsorption and levels, possibly leading to toxicity. Toxic effects may include ventricular arrhythmias, cinchonism (headache, palpitations, dizziness, visual disturbances, tinnitus).

Suggestions: Advise patients to:

Favor acidifying foods: bread, bacon, corn, lentils, meat, fish, fowl, cranberries, plums, prunes.

Minimize or avoid alkalinizing foods: milk and other dairy products, vegetables, almonds, chestnuts, coconuts, citrus juices.

Also advise patients to promptly report any toxic symptoms.

Note: Quinine (#862) is chemically related to quinidine and may react the same way.

FOODS   ⟷   THYROID HORMONES

214   886

Reaction: Certain foods contain goitrogens, which exacerbate any existent thyroid deficiency.

Suggestion: Advise patients on thyroid replacement therapy to avoid the following goitrogenic foods: leafy green vegetables (asparagus, broccoli, Brussels sprouts, cabbage, kale, lettuce, peas, spinach, turnip greens, watercress); soy beans.

FOODS   ⟷   TETRACYCLINES

240   416
386   880

Reaction: All foods, but especially milk and other dairy products, significantly decrease the oral absorption of all tetracyclines except minocycline (#386, no interference) and doxycycline (#240, minimal interference).

Decreased tetracycline absorption (with the above exceptions) also occurs with antacids, iron preparations, vitamin-mineral preparations, and laxatives with magnesium (eg, Epsom salts, milk of magnesia).

Suggestions: Give tetracyclines 1 hour before or 2 hours after meals.

For maximal therapeutic effect and patient compliance, it may be best to prescribe a tetracycline preparation that can be taken only one or two times a day (eg, minocycline, doxycycline). Unfortunately, cost factors may outweigh this consideration.

F-17

FOODS   ⟷   **CALCIUM CARBONATE/SODIUM BICARBONATE**

500   726

Reaction: The consumption of large quantities of milk or dairy products along with calcium carbonate or sodium bicarbonate over prolonged periods can produce a "milk-alkali syndrome" of hypercalcemia, with abdominal pain, anorexia, nausea, vomiting, diarrhea, possible muscle weakness. Irreversible renal damage can occur from precipitation of calcium salts in the renal parenchyma.

Suggestion: Avoid.

F-18

FOODS   ⟷   **CAPTOPRIL**

616

Reaction: Foods reduce the absorption of captopril.

Suggestion: Give captopril approximately 1 hour before meals.

F-19

FOODS   ⟷   **DIGOXIN**

224

Reaction: Possible decreased absorption of digoxin if taken simultaneously with bran cereal or other high-fiber foods (bran, whole wheat, grains, fruits, raw vegetables, leafy cooked vegetables).

Suggestions: Give digoxin ½ hour before or 2 hours after high-fiber foods.

Appendix: Generic Names by Number

HOW TO USE THIS SECTION

The APPENDIX converts drug code numbers into generic names. (Common trade names for each generic name can be found in Section I: NAME INDEX.)

Drugs that react identically have identical code numbers. For example, #788 represents eight different cephalosporin-type antibacterials, all of which participate in the same interactions. But a number of cephalosporins have unique interactions of their own. As a result, there are five other code numbers (160, 162, 164, 590, 618) for additional cephalosporins that are not listed in the #788 group.

The APPENDIX also provides a brief description of the clinical orientation and use of each drug or drug class.

102 acetaminophen
—Analgesic; antipyretic

104 acetazolamide
—Carbonic anhydrase inhibitor; anticonvulsant; reduces intraocular pressure in glaucoma

106 actinomycin D (dactinomycin)
—Antineoplastic

108 alcohol
—Mood elevator in small doses (by suppressing inhibitions); sedative-depressant in larger doses

110 allopurinol
—Antigout

112 aluminum aspirin
aspirin
calcium carbaspirin
—Aspirin-type analgesics and antipyretics

114 amantadine
—Antiparkinsonian; antiviral

116 para-aminobenzoic acid (aminobenzoic acid, PABA)
—Topical sunburn protectant (sunscreen); considered member of vitamin B complex; used orally as dietary supplement

118 para-aminosalicylic acid (aminosalicylic acid, P.A.S.)
—Antitubercular

120 amphotericin B
—Antifungal; antiprotozoal

122 ampicillin
bacampicillin
—Antibacterials (penicillin-type)

124 antimony potassium tartrate
—Antischistosomiasis

126 antipyrine
—Analgesic; antipyretic

128 ascorbic acid (vitamin C)
—Antiscurvy vitamin

130 asparaginase
—Antineoplastic

132 atropine
—Anticholinergic antispasmodic; antiarrhythmic; mydriatic and cycloplegic (dilates pupil and paralyzes accommodation)

134 azathioprine
—Antineoplastic

136 belladonna alkaloids, extract, leaf, or tincture (hyoscyamine)
—Anticholinergic antispasmodic

138 benzphetamine
—Appetite suppressant; CNS stimulant

140 dicumarol (bishydroxycoumarin)
—Anticoagulant

142 blood from blood bank
—Possible factor in hyperkalemia

144 busulfan
—Antineoplastic

146 caffeine
—Xanthine; appetite suppressant; CNS stimulant; bronchodilator

148 capreomycin
—Antitubercular

150 carbamazepine
—Anticonvulsant; sedative for trigeminal neuralgia

152 carbenicillin
—Antibacterial (penicillin-type)

154 carbenoxolone
—Steroid-like licorice ingredient with anti-inflammatory and aldosterone-like activity; used in treatment of peptic ulcer

156 carisoprodol
—Skeletal muscle relaxant

158 carmustine (BCNU)
—Antineoplastic

160 cephaloridine
—Antibacterial (cephalosporin-type)

162 cephalothin
—Antibacterial (cephalosporin-type)

164 cephradine
—Antibacterial (cephalosporin-type)

166 chloramphenicol
—Antibacterial

168 chlordiazepoxide
—Sedative-hypnotic (benzodiazepine-type); minor (antianxiety) tranquilizer

170 chlorphenesin
—Skeletal muscle relaxant

172 chlorphenoxamine
—Anticholinergic with central (antidyskinetic) activity

174 chlorpromazine
—Sedative-hypnotic (phenothiazine-type); major (antipsychotic) tranquilizer

176 chlorpropamide
—Oral hypoglycemic

178 cholestyramine
—Antihyperlipidemic; antidiarrheal

180 cimetidine
—Histamine H_2 receptor antagonist; used in treatment of peptic ulcer

182 cisplatin
—Antineoplastic

184 clindamycin
—Antibacterial

186 clofibrate
—Antihyperlipidemic

188 clonazepam
—Sedative-hypnotic (benzodiazepine-type); minor (antianxiety) tranquilizer

190 clonidine
—Antihypertensive

192 codeine
—Narcotic analgesic

194 colestipol
—Antihyperlipidemic

196 colistimethate
—Antibacterial (polymyxin-type)

198 colistin (polymyxin E)
— Antibacterial
(polymyxin-type)
200 corticotropin
— Adrenal cortex-
stimulating hormone
202 hydrocortisone (cortisol)
— Corticosteroid
(glucocorticoid and
mineralocorticoid)
204 cyclophosphamide
— Antineoplastic
206 cycloserine
— Antitubercular
208 dapsone
— Antileprosy
210 desoxycorticosterone
— Corticosteroid
(mineralocorticoid)
212 dextromethorphan
— Antitussive
214 dextrothyroxine
— Antihyperlipidemic
216 diazepam
— Sedative-hypnotic
(benzodiazepine-type);
minor (antianxiety)
tranquilizer
218 diazoxide
— Antihypertensive
220 dicyclomine
— Anticholinergic
antispasmodic
222 digitoxin
— Digitalis glycoside
224 digoxin
— Digitalis glycoside
226 diphenhydramine
— Antihistamine
228 diphenoxylate
— Antiperistaltic
antidiarrheal

230 disopyramide
— Antiarrhythmic
232 disulfiram
— Antialcoholic
234 dopamine
— Adrenergic;
vasopressor; used in
treatment of shock
236 doxapram
— Appetite suppressant;
CNS stimulant;
respiratory stimulant
238 doxorubicin
— Antineoplastic
240 doxycycline
— Antibacterial
(tetracycline-type)
242 droperidol
— Major tranquilizer;
used principally as
anesthetic or
preanesthetic agent
244 echothiophate
— Miotic (constricts
pupil); used in
glaucoma
246 edrophonium
— Parasympathomimetic
(cholinergic); used in
abdominal
hypoperistalsis,
neurogenic urinary
retention, myasthenia
gravis
248 ephedrine
— Adrenergic
250 epinephrine
— Adrenergic
252 erythromycin estolate
— Antibacterial
(erythromycin-type)
254 ethacrynic acid
— Diuretic

256 ethchlorvynol
—Sedative-hypnotic;
minor tranquilizer;
used to treat agitation,
anxiety, insomnia

258 ethinamate
—Sedative-hypnotic;
minor tranquilizer;
used to treat agitation,
anxiety, insomnia

260 ethopropazine
—Anticholinergic with
central (antidyskinetic)
activity

262 fenfluramine
—Appetite suppressant;
CNS *depressant* (all
other appetite
suppressants are CNS
stimulants)

264 fentanyl
—Narcotic analgesic

266 fludrocortisone
—Corticosteroid
(mineralocorticoid)

268 flunitrazepam
—Sedative-hypnotic
(benzodiazepine-type);
minor (antianxiety)
tranquilizer

270 fluroxene
—General inhalation
anesthetic

272 folic acid
—B complex vitamin
used in various types of
anemia

274 furazolidone
—Antibacterial
(nitrofurantoin-type);
also has monoamine
oxidase inhibitor
(antidepressant) activity

276 furosemide
—Diuretic

278 gentamicin
—Antibacterial
(aminoglycoside-type)

280 glucagon
—Used to treat insulin
shock (metabolizes liver
glycogen to raise blood
sugar)

282 glutethimide
—Sedative-hypnotic; used
principally for its
hypnotic effect

284 glycopyrrolate
—Anticholinergic with
both central
(antidyskinetic) and
peripheral
(antispasmodic) activity

288 griseofulvin
—Antifungal

290 haloperidol
—Antipsychotic sedative;
major tranquilizer

292 halothane
—General inhalation
anesthetic

294 heparin
—Anticoagulant

296 hydralazine
—Antihypertensive

298 hydroxyzine
—Antihistamine

300 ibuprofen
—Nonsteroidal anti-
inflammatory

302 indomethacin
—Nonsteroidal anti-
inflammatory

304 insulin
—Antidiabetic

366 methohexital
—Sedative-hypnotic
(barbiturate-type);
minor (antianxiety)
tranquilizer; also used
for general anesthesia

368 methotrexate
—Antineoplastic

370 methotrimeprazine
—Narcotic analgesic

372 methoxyflurane
—General inhalation
anesthetic

374 methscopolamine
—Anticholinergic
antispasmodic

376 methyldopa
—Antihypertensive

378 methylphenidate
—Appetite suppressant;
CNS stimulant; also
used for treatment of
hyperkinesis

380 metoclopramide
—Antiemetic; stimulates
motility of upper GI
tract

382 metoprolol
—Beta blocker
(antianginal,
antiarrhythmic,
antihypertensive)

384 metronidazole
—Anthelmintic;
antiprotozoal

386 minocycline
—Antibacterial
(tetracycline-type)

388 minoxidil
—Antihypertensive

390 morphine
—Narcotic analgesic

392 nadolol
—Beta blocker
(antianginal,
antiarrhythmic,
antihypertensive)

394 nalidixic acid
—Urinary tract
antibacterial

396 neomycin
—Antibacterial
(aminoglycoside-type)

398 niacin (nicotinic acid)
—Antihyperlipidemic;
antipellagra vitamin

400 nitrofurantoin
—Urinary tract
antibacterial

402 nitroglycerin
—Antianginal; coronary
artery dilator

404 norethindrone
—Progestogen hormone

406 opium alkaloids
—Narcotic analgesic

408 orphenadrine
—Skeletal muscle
relaxant

410 oxacillin
—Antibacterial
(penicillin-type)

412 oxycodone
—Narcotic analgesic

414 oxyphenbutazone
—Nonsteroidal anti-
inflammatory

416 oxytetracycline
—Antibacterial
(tetracycline-type)

418 papaverine
—Peripheral vasodilator

420 paraldehyde
—Sedative-hypnotic

422 penicillin G potassium
—Antibacterial
(penicillin-type)

424 penicillin V potassium
—Antibacterial
(penicillin-type)

428 pentazocine
—Narcotic analgesic

430 pentobarbital
—Sedative-hypnotic
(barbiturate-type);
minor (antianxiety)
tranquilizer; anesthetic

432 phenacetin
—Analgesic; antipyretic

434 phenobarbital
—Sedative-hypnotic
(barbiturate-type);
minor (antianxiety)
tranquilizer

436 phenoxybenzamine
—Alpha blocker; used in
prostatism and as
antihypertensive in
pheochromocytoma

438 phentolamine
—Adrenergic blocker;
used as
antihypertensive in
pheochromocytoma

440 phenylbutazone
—Nonsteroidal anti-
inflammatory

442 phenylephrine
—Adrenergic; used
principally as a nasal
decongestant

444 phenylpropanolamine
—Adrenergic; used
principally as a nasal
decongestant

446 phenytoin
—Anticonvulsant
(hydantoin-type);
antiarrhythmic

450 polymyxin B sulfate
—Antibacterial
(polymyxin-type)

452 prazosin
—Antihypertensive

456 primidone
—Anticonvulsant

458 probenecid
—Uricosuric

460 procainamide
—Antiarrhythmic

462 procaine
—Local anesthetic

464 procarbazine
—Antineoplastic; also has
monoamine oxidase
inhibitor
(antidepressant) activity

466 prochlorperazine
—Sedative-hypnotic
(phenothiazine-type);
major (antipsychotic)
tranquilizer

468 promazine
—Sedative-hypnotic
(phenothiazine-type);
major (antipsychotic)
tranquilizer

470 propantheline
—Anticholinergic
antispasmodic

472 propiomazine
—Sedative-hypnotic
(phenothiazine-type);
major (antipsychotic)
tranquilizer

474 propoxyphene
—Narcotic analgesic

476 propranolol
— Beta blocker (antianginal, antiarrhythmic, antihypertensive)

478 propylthiouracil
— Antihyperthyroid

480 protokylol
— Adrenergic

482 pyridoxine (vitamin B$_6$)
— Anti-anemia vitamin; used in some neurological diseases, dermatoses, nausea and vomiting of pregnancy

484 pyrimethamine
— Antimalarial

486 quinacrine
— Anthelmintic; antimalarial

488 radiation therapy
— Cause of myelosuppression

490 rifampin
— Antitubercular

492 scopolamine (hyoscine)
— Anticholinergic; used principally as preanesthetic agent and for motion sickness

494 secobarbital
— Sedative-hypnotic (barbiturate-type); minor (antianxiety) tranquilizer

496 smallpox and other live vaccines
— Cause of generalized vaccinia

498 sodium acid phosphate (sodium biphosphate)
— Urinary acidifier

500 sodium bicarbonate
— Antacid; urinary alkalinizer

502 sodium chloride
— Electrolyte

504 sodium nitroprusside
— Antihypertensive

506 sodium polystyrene sulfonate resin
— Potassium exchange resin

508 spironolactone
— Potassium-sparing diuretic

510 streptomycin
— Antibacterial (aminoglycoside-type)

512 succinylcholine
— Curare-like neuromuscular blocker

514 sulfamethizole
— Antibacterial (sulfonamide-type)

516 sulfamethoxazole
— Antibacterial (sulfonamide-type)

522 sulfasalazine
— Antibacterial (sulfonamide-type)

524 sulfinpyrazone
— Antibacterial (sulfonamide-type)

526 sulfisoxazole
— Antibacterial (sulfonamide-type)

530 thiamylal
— Sedative-hypnotic (barbiturate-type); minor (antianxiety) tranquilizer; general anesthetic

532 thiopental
—Sedative-hypnotic
(barbiturate-type);
general anesthetic

534 thiotepa
—Antineoplastic

536 ticarcillin
—Antibacterial
(penicillin-type)

538 tobramycin
—Antibacterial
(aminoglycoside-type)

540 tocopherol (vitamin E)
—Used topically for skin
care; other uses
currently controversial

542 tolazoline
—Peripheral vasodilator

544 tolbutamide
—Oral hypoglycemic

546 triamterene
—Potassium-sparing
diuretic

548 triclofos
—Sedative-hypnotic;
minor tranquilizer;
used to treat agitation,
anxiety, insomnia

550 trihexyphenidyl
—Anticholinergic with
central (antidyskinetic)
activity

552 trimethadione
—Anticonvulsant

554 trimethobenzamide
—Antiemetic

556 troleandomycin
—Antibacterial

558 valproic acid
—Anticonvulsant

560 vancomycin
—Antibacterial

562 vincristine
—Antineoplastic

564 viomycin
—Antitubercular

566 vitamin D
—Antirachitic; calcium
regulator

568 warfarin
—Anticoagulant

570 zinc sulfate
—Ophthalmological
antiseptic; emetic

572 megestrol
—Progestogen hormone

574 penicillamine
—Heavy metal chelating
agent

576 norgestrel
—Progestogen hormone

580 bethanechol
—Parasympathomimetic
(cholinergic); used in
abdominal
hypoperistalsis,
neurogenic urinary
retention, myasthenia
gravis

582 carbromal
—Sedative-hypnotic;
minor (antianxiety)
tranquilizer

584 diethylstilbestrol
—Estrogenic hormone

586 medroxyprogesterone
—Progestogen hormone

588 hexobarbital
—Sedative-hypnotic
(barbiturate-type);
minor (antianxiety)
tranquilizer

590 moxalactam
—Antibacterial
(cephalosporin-type)

592 metaproterenol
—Adrenergic

594 methoxyphenamine
—Adrenergic

596 pseudoephedrine
—Adrenergic; used
principally as a nasal
decongestant

598 terbutaline
—Adrenergic; used
principally for
bronchodilation

600 methimazole
—Antihyperthyroid

602 ethylnorepinephrine
—Adrenergic

604 isoetharine
—Adrenergic; used
principally for
bronchodilation

606 sulindac
—Nonsteroidal anti-
inflammatory

608 influenza vaccine
—Cause of theophylline
toxicity

610 vidarabine
—Antiviral

612 vitamin A
—Necessary for growth
and bone development
in children; normal
vision and epithelial
integrity in adults

614 amiloride
—Potassium-sparing
diuretic

616 captopril
—Antihypertensive

618 cefamandole
—Antibacterial
(cephalosporin-type)

620 sucralfate
—Forms protein complex
that coats and protects
duodenal ulcers from
acid and pepsin

702 activated charcoal
attapulgite
kaolin
pectin
—Adsorbents

704 amikacin
kanamycin
—Antibacterials
(aminoglycoside-type)

706 amphetamine
dextroamphetamine
methamphetamine
*pemoline
—Amphetamines
*A closely related
compound

708 danazol
ethylestrenol
methandrostenolone
nandrolone
norethandrolone
oxandrolone
oxymetholone
stanozolol
—Anabolic steroids; used
to stimulate metabolism
in debilitated patients

712 calusterone
dromostanolone
fluoxymesterone
methyltestosterone
testolactone
testosterone
—Androgenic steroids;
used in hypogonadism,
delayed puberty,
metastatic breast
carcinoma

714 ketamine
—General anesthetic
716 cyclopropane
enflurane
ether
isoflurane
nitrous oxide
—General inhalation
anesthetics
718 benzocaine
butacaine
cyclomethycaine
dibucaine
hexylcaine
tetracaine
—Local anesthetics;
derivatives of para-
aminobenzoic acid
722 aluminum carbonate gel
aluminum glycinate
aluminum hydroxide
aluminum phosphate
dihydroxyaluminum
aminoacetate
dihydroxyaluminum
sodium carbonate
—Aluminum-containing
antacids
726 calcium carbonate
—Calcium-containing
antacid
728 magnesium trisilicate
—Magnesium-containing
antacid
730 amyl nitrite
dipyridamole
erythrityl tetranitrate
mannitol hexanitrate
pentaerythritol
tetranitrate
—Antianginal agents
732 bretylium
—Antiarrhythmic

736 benztropine
biperiden
caramiphen
carbetapentane
cyclopentolate
cycrimine
procyclidine
—Anticholinergics with
central (antidyskinetic)
activity; used for
treatment of various
motion disorders—
parkinsonism,
epilepsy, etc.
738 anisotropine
benactyzine
clidinium
diphemanil
flavoxate
hexocyclium
homatropine
mepenzolate
methantheline
methixene
oxybutynin
oxyphencyclimine
oxyphenonium
thiphenamil
tridihexethyl
—Anticholinergic
antispasmodics
(anticholinergics with
peripheral activity)
742 phenprocoumon
—Anticoagulant
744 anisindione
phenindione
—Anticoagulants
(indanedione
derivatives)
746 paramethadione
phenacemide
—Anticonvulsants

770 *(continued)*
    phendimetrazine
    phenmetrazine
    phentermine
    —Appetite suppressants;
      CNS stimulants
772 allobarbital
    amobarbital
    aprobarbital
    barbital
    butabarbital
    butalbital
    mephobarbital
    metharbital
    talbutal
    —Sedative-hypnotics
      (barbiturate-type);
      minor (antianxiety)
      tranquilizers
774 alprazolam
    clorazepate
    flurazepam
    halazepam
    lorazepam
    nitrazepam
    oxazepam
    prazepam
    temazepam
    —Sedative-hypnotics
      (benzodiazepine-type);
      minor (antianxiety)
      tranquilizers
776 atenolol
    timolol
    —Beta blockers
      (antianginal,
      antiarrhythmic
      antihypertensive)
778 calcium chloride
    calcium gluceptate
    calcium gluconate
    calcium lactate
      continued

778 *(continued)*
    —Calcium-replacement
      preparations, parenteral
780 chlormezanone
    tybamate
    —Sedative-hypnotics
      (carbamate-type);
      minor (antianxiety)
      tranquilizers
782 dichlorphenamide
    ethoxzolamide
    methazolamide
    —Carbonic anhydrase
      inhibitors; reduce
      intraocular pressure in
      glaucoma
784 methyprylon
    —CNS depressant; used
      principally for its
      hypnotic effect
786 deanol
    pentylenetetrazol
    —CNS stimulants;
      appetite suppressants
788 cefaclor
    cefadroxil
    cefazolin
    cefotaxime
    cefoxitin
    cephalexin
    cephaloglycin
    cephapirin
    —Antibacterials
      (cephalosporin-type)
790 chloral betaine
    chloral hydrate
    —Sedative-hypnotics
      (chloral derivatives);
      used to treat agitation,
      anxiety, insomnia
792 acetylcholine chloride
    ambenonium
      continued

818 aurothioglucose
gold sodium thiomalate
—Gold salts; used as
nonsteroidal anti-
inflammatory agents
820 guanethidine
—Antihypertensive
822 BCG (tuberculosis
vaccine)
dantrolene (skeletal
muscle relaxant)
ethionamide
(antitubercular)
phenazopyridine (urinary
tract analgesic)
pyrazinamide
(antitubercular)
thiabendazole
(anthelmintic)
—Potential hepatotoxins
824 ethotoin
mephenytoin
—Anticonvulsants
(hydantoin-type)
826 acetohexamide
tolazamide
—Oral hypoglycemics
828 calcium iodide
hydriodic acid
iodinated glycerol
potassium iodide
strong iodine solution
—Iodine-containing
compounds
830 ferrocholinate
ferrous fumarate
ferrous gluconate
ferrous sulfate
iron
iron bile salts
iron-polysaccharide
complex
—Iron preparations

832 barley malt extract
bisacodyl
cascara sagrada
castor oil
danthron
docusate (dioctyl sodium
sulfosuccinate)
methylcellulose
mineral oil
phenolphthalein
psyllium
senna
—Laxatives
834 magnesium citrate
magnesium sulfate—oral
—Laxatives
836 isocarboxazid
pargyline
phenelzine
tranylcypromine
—Antidepressants
(monoamine oxidase
inhibitors)
838 flucytosine (antifungal)
idoxuridine (antiviral)
sulfoxone (antileprosy)
suramin (antiprotozoal)
—Myelosuppressants
840 alphaprodine
anileridine
butorphanol
ethoheptazine
hydrocodone
hydromorphone
levorphanol
nalbuphine
oxymorphone
—Narcotic analgesics
844 methicillin
nafcillin—injection
penicillin G benzathine—
injection
continued

844 *(continued)*
    penicillin G procaine
    penicillin V benzathine
    —Parenteral penicillins

846 amoxicillin
    cloxacillin
    cyclacillin
    dicloxacillin
    hetacillin
    nafcillin—oral
    penicillin G benzathine—
       oral
    penicillin V
    —Oral penicillins

848 acetophenazine
    butaperazine
    carphenazine
    fluphenazine
    mesoridazine
    perphenazine
    piperacetazine
    thiethylperazine
    thiopropazate
    thioridazine
    trifluoperazine
    triflupromazine
    —Sedative-hypnotics
      (phenothiazine-type);
      major (antipsychotic)
      tranquilizers

854 salt substitutes containing
      potassium
    —Possible factor in
      hyperkalemia

856 potassium acetate
    potassium bicarbonate
    potassium chloride
    potassium citrate
    potassium gluconate
    —Potassium preparations

860 dimethisterone
    dydrogesterone
    ethisterone
    ethynodiol diacetate
    hydroxyprogesterone
    norethynodrel
    progesterone
    —Progestogen hormones

862 quinidine
    *quinine
    —Antiarrhythmic
    *A closely related
    antimalarial compound

864 alseroxylon
    deserpidine
    rauwolfia serpentina
      (whole root rauwolfia)
    rescinnamine
    reserpine
    syrosingopine
    —Antihypertensives
      (reserpine and related
      drugs)

866 bismuth subsalicylate
    choline salicylate
    magnesium salicylate
    phenyl salicylate
    potassium salicylate
    salicylamide
    salsalate
    sodium salicylate
    sodium thiosalicylate
    —Salicylates

868 baclofen
    chlorzoxazone
    cyclobenzaprine
    mephenesin
    metaxalone
    —Skeletal muscle
      relaxants with central
      (CNS) activity

870 ethosuximide
methsuximide
phensuximide
—Anticonvulsants
(succinimides)

872 mafenide
sulfabenzamide
sulfacetamide
sulfacytine
sulfadiazine
sulfamerazine
sulfameter
sulfamethazine
sulfanilamide
sulfapyridine
sulfathiazole
—Antibacterials
(sulfonamide-type)

876 albuterol
dobutamine
methoxamine
naphazoline
oxymetazoline
propylhexedrine
tetrahydrozoline
xylometazoline
—Direct-acting
adrenergics
(sympathomimetics);
act directly on effector
cells rather than via
release of
norepinephrine

878 cyclopentamine
mephentermine*
racephedrine
—Indirect-acting
adrenergics (sympatho-
mimetics); cause release
of norepinephrine,
which in turn acts on
effector cells
continued

878 *(continued)*
*Mephentermine is
both direct- and
indirect-acting.

880 chlortetracycline
demeclocycline
methacycline
tetracycline
—Antibacterials
(tetracycline-type)

882 bendroflumethiazide
benzthiazide
chlorothiazide
*chlorthalidone
cyclothiazide
flumethiazide
hydrochlorothiazide
hydroflumethiazide
methyclothiazide
*metolazone
polythiazide
*quinethazone
trichlormethiazide
—Diuretics
(thiazide-type)
*Closely related
compounds

884 chlorprothixene
thiothixene
—Sedative-hypnotics
(thioxanthene-type);
major (antipsychotic)
tranquilizers

886 levothyroxine
liothyronine
liotrix
thyroglobulin
thyroid
—Thyroid-type hormones

888 amitriptyline
amoxapine
desipramine
continued

888 *(continued)*
doxepin
imipramine
maprotiline
nortriptyline
protriptyline
trimipramine
—Tricyclic
antidepressants; have
tranquilizing effect that
relieves depression
(mood elevators in
small doses; depressants
in larger doses)

890 tyramine-containing foods
(see list in Food
Interaction #F-6)

892 ammonium acid
phosphate
ammonium chloride
hippuric acid
potassium acid phosphate
sodium acid
pyrophosphate
—Urinary acidifiers

896 cyclandelate
dioxyline phosphate
ethaverine
isoxsuprine
nicotinyl alcohol
nylidrin
—Peripheral vasodilators

898 menadiol sodium
(vitamin K_4)
menadione (vitamin K_3)
phytonadione
(vitamin K_1)
—Vitamin K; blood-
clotting agents

902 aminophylline
dyphylline
oxtriphylline
theophylline
—Xanthines; used
principally for
bronchodilation

910 nifedipine
verapamil
—Calcium blockers; used
as antiarrhythmics

Bibliography

The following sources, listed alphabetically, are recommended for further information on drug therapy and interactions:

1. **AMA DRUG EVALUATIONS.**
   4th edition, 1980. Prepared by the AMA Department of Drugs; published by the American Medical Association, Chicago, Ill.; distributed by John Wiley & Sons, Inc., 605 Third Ave., New York, N.Y. 10158.
   —General information on drug use, precautions, indications, and complications.

2. **CLIN-ALERT.**
   Published biweekly by Science Editors, Inc., 149 Thierman Lane, Louisville, Ky. 40207.
   —Excellent source for up-to-date information, especially on side effects.

3. **DRUG INTERACTIONS.**
   4th edition, 1979. By Philip D. Hansten, Pharm.D. Published by Lea & Febiger, 600 S. Washington Square, Philadelphia, Pa. 19106.
   —Best-referenced source for interactions; relative importance of interactions indicated graphically.

4. **DRUG INTERACTIONS NEWSLETTER.**
   Edited by Philip D. Hansten, Pharm.D. Published monthly by Applied Therapeutics, Inc., P.O. Box 31-747, San Francisco, Calif. 94131.
   —Up-to-date information on interactions.

5. **EVALUATIONS OF DRUG INTERACTIONS.**
   2nd edition, 1976. Prepared and published by the American Pharmaceutical Association, 2215 Constitution Ave., N.W., Washington, D.C. 20037. Supplement published in 1978.
   —Detailed discussions extrapolating results from specific to related drugs.

6. **THE MEDICAL LETTER.**
   Published biweekly by The Medical Letter, Inc., a nonprofit corporation, 56 Harrison St., New Rochelle, N.Y. 10801.
   —*Most readable source for the average physician concerning new drug developments.*

7. **UNITED STATES PHARMACOPEIA DISPENSING INFORMATION, 1981.**
   Published by the United States Pharmacopeial Convention, Inc., U.S.P. Drug Information Division, Publications Department, 12601 Twinbrook Parkway, Rockville, Md. 20852. Revised approximately every 15 months; updates issued bimonthly.
   —*Good source for translating medical to lay terminology, and for dispensing information and precautions; relative importance of interactions indicated graphically.*